Dedication

To my teachers, especially
Roman W. Desanctis and Saul J. Farber

Contents

Preface

Cardiac arrhythmias are among our most common afflictions. Usually they have little clinical importance and present no risk to the life of patients who have them. Occasionally, however, they can produce troublesome symptoms and may even bring about the patient's death.*

Arrhythmias produce rapid, slow, or irregular heartbeats of which some patients may be acutely conscious, whereas others may be unaware. Explaining what arrhythmias are and how doctors treat them—when that is necessary—is the purpose of this book.

First I explain the anatomy and physiology of the heart, particularly of the electrical components that give rise to arrhythmias.

Then I describe most of the arrhythmias that patients may develop. Each chapter has been built around the experiences of a patient for whom the author or one his colleagues has cared. In some cases, I have changed the stories slightly to facilitate understanding and to avoid confusing the picture with issues that the doctors might have needed to consider but are unrelated to the topic being discussed. In the next section, I explain how cardiologists use drugs and

---

* For a more comprehensive discussion of the subject, some readers may want to consult the author's text *Arrhythmias* (Philadelphia, W.B. Saunders, 2000).

devices such as pacemakers and implantable defibrillators to treat arrhythmias.

I then invite the reader to take a short course in electrocardiography, for it is this familiar test that we use to diagnose arrhythmias and evaluate the effects of treatment. The reader will find electrocardiograms of some of the arrhythmias discussed in the case reports to see how cardiologists recognize which arrhythmia is which.

The analysis of arrhythmias has, in recent decades, become so complex that a subspecialty of cardiology has developed for those who study this subject. Some call the practitioners of this art *arrhythmologists*, a name that no reader of this book is required to learn. Many arrhythmologists work in cardiac electrophysiology laboratories, large rooms filled with electronic computerized equipment where the details of patients' arrhythmias are studied and appropriate treatments are planned and instituted. By describing what goes on in these laboratories, I will try to relieve some of the concern that patients who undergo these procedures may have and dispel some of the mystery about what those working in these laboratories are doing.

It is difficult to describe all medical conditions without using some of the terms that we learn in medical school. Most of those used in this book are listed in the glossary. In case you forget some of them, I have repeated the definitions of many in the text.

As a break from all of this medicalese, I have added two historical vignettes of doctors who have made important contributions to the field of arrhythmias. The first tells the extraordinary story of the man who invented the implantable cardioverter defibrillator, one of the most important advances in cardiology in recent decades. The second describes the contributions of three men, two American and one British, who first described an arrhythmia that now bears their names.

I thank Dr. Eric Rashba, my colleague at the University of Maryland, who read the entire manuscript and made several important suggestions to improve the accuracy of the text. Wendy Goodwin, director of our electrocardiogram laboratory, helped me collect many of the tracings. Phyllis Farrell, executive secretary in the Department of Medicine at Maryland, read the proof and, as in my previous books, picked up several mistakes that I had missed. My wife Mae read the revised proof and suggested several important changes that clarified some of my more obtuse explanations. Thanks Phyllis and Mae.

Readers of the *New England Journal of Medicine* will recognize the general construction of the cases—the clinical information presented first (shaded box) followed by the discussions—as similar in appearance to the "Clinical Practice" articles in that journal.

At Jones and Bartlett, I thank Christopher Davis, Executive Publisher for Medicine, Kathy Richardson, Associate Editor, Kate Hennessy from production, and Laura Kavigian from marketing.

John A. Kastor
Baltimore, MD

Glossary of Medical Terms and Definitions

Medical Terms	Definitions and Derivation
Aorta	The largest artery through which all blood destined for the body, except the lungs, leaves the heart.
Aortic valve	Prevents blood flowing backward from the aorta to the left ventricle.
Arteries	Vessels carrying blood from the heart to the body and from the right ventricle to the lungs.
Atria	Smaller heart chambers receiving blood from the body and the lungs and delivering it to the ventricles ("Atrium," plural "atria," = the central room in a Roman house).
Atrioventricular (A-V) node	The conducting tissue in the floor of the right atrium that electrically links the atria to the bundle of His and delays conduction briefly to allow the ventricles to contract most efficiently.

Autonomic nervous system	A neurological system that is not under conscious control.
Bradycardia	Slow heart rate.
Bundle branches	Collections of conducting tissue that carry the electrical impulse from the bundle of His to the ventricles.
Bundle of His	Conducting tissue between the atrioventricular node and the bundle branches.
Cardiomyopathy	Disease of the heart muscle.
Diastole	Relaxation phase of the heart chambers.
Dilate	Enlarge.
Diuretic	Drug that induces production of urine.
Dyspnea	Breathlessness, shortness of breath.
Echocardiogram	The clinical device that records the size and function of the cardiac chambers and valves.
Edema	Fluid collected in the legs, lungs, and other organs in patients with congestive heart failure.
Ejection fraction	A measurement of the ability of the ventricles to eject blood.
Electrocardiogram	The clinical device that records the electrical activity of the heart.
Emboli	Blood clots released into the circulation.
Endocardium	Inner lining of the heart, usually used in reference to the ventricles.
Insufficiency	Leaking of a cardiac valve.
Ischemia	The effect of insufficient blood supply to the heart muscle.
Lone	Without known cause.
Mitral valve	Prevents blood from flowing backward from the left ventricle to the left atrium (has two cusps or leaflets;

	derived from *miter*, the liturgical headdress worn by a bishop that has two spade-like parts).
Palpitations	The sensation of irregularities in the heartbeat.
Parasympathetic	One of the functional divisions of the autonomic nervous system.
Paroxysm	Episode.
Polyuria	Much urine.
Premature	Early (as in premature beats).
Pulmonary	Relating to the lung.
Pulmonary valve	Prevents blood from flowing backward from the pulmonary arteries to the right ventricle.
Pulse deficit	The difference in the heart rate as detected by listening to the heart and feeling a peripheral pulse.
Purkinje fibers	Network of conducting tissue lining the endocardium of the ventricles.
Regurgitation	Leaking of a cardiac valve.
Sinus or sinoatrial (SA) node	The primary pacemaker of the heart, located in the right atrium near the superior vena cava ("sinus" = curve, fold, or hollow; "node" = knot [of tissue]).
Stenosis	Narrowing (as in the opening of the cardiac valves).
Superior vena cava	The large vein draining the upper part of the body (translation: "upper hollow vein").
Sympathetic	One of the functional divisions of the autonomic nervous system.
Symptom	Medical complaint.
Syncope	Fainting, losing consciousness.
Systole	Contraction phase of the heart chambers.

Tachycardia	Rapid heart rate.
Tricuspid valve	Prevents blood from flowing backward from the right ventricle to the right atrium (has three cusps or leaflets).
Vagus nerve	An important nerve of the parasympathetic nervous system that takes a long and circuitous path from the brain to the other organs of the body that it affects. "Vagus" = wandering.
Veins	Vessels carrying blood from the body to the heart and from the lungs to the left atrium.
Ventricles	Two larger heart chambers each receiving blood from the atria. The right ventricle delivers blood to the lungs, the left to the body.

Part I

How the Heart Works

Chapter 1

The Heart as a Pump

The heart's fundamental function is pumping blood through the body. This process is coordinated by an electrical system within the heart that, when it malfunctions, produces arrhythmias.

First, some anatomy and physiology. The heart in humans is a hollow muscular organ with four chambers, two atria and two ventricles (Figure 1-1). From the picture, let us follow the route of the blood as it courses through the chambers of the heart (Figure 1-2). Blood from most of the veins of the body enters the right atrium, which ejects the blood into the right ventricle past the tricuspid valve. From here the blood is propelled past the pulmonary valve through the pulmonary arteries and into the lungs. The oxygenated blood is collected from the lungs in the pulmonary veins and enters the left atrium, where it is passes through the mitral valve into the left ventricle, the heart's principal pumping chamber. The left ventricle then pumps the blood past the aortic valve to the arteries, which distribute the blood to the rest of the body. The tricuspid and mitral valves prevent the blood from being ejected backward into the atria, and the pulmonary and aortic valves (semilunar valves) prevent regurgitation into the ventricles. The *endocardium* lines the chambers, the

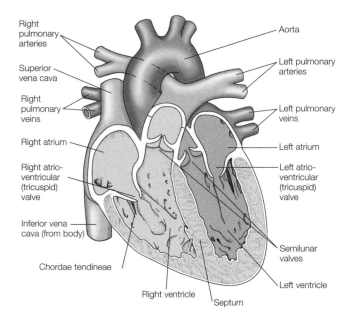

FIGURE 1-1   Anatomy of the Heart

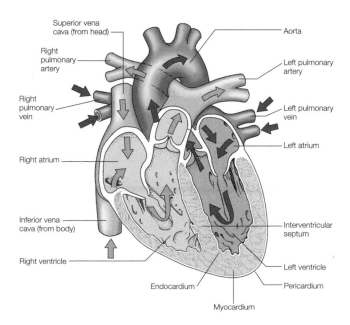

FIGURE 1-2   Blood Flow Through the Heart

myocardium is the heart muscle, and the *pericardium* is a sac that surrounds the heart. Blood from the upper part of the body enters the right atrium through the *superior vena cava* and from the rest of the body through the *inferior vena cava*. The *interventricular septum* separates the two ventricles. The *chordae tendineae* are fibrous cords that connect the mitral and triscuspid valves to the myocardium.

The muscles lining the chambers contract and relax. During contraction (*systole*), the blood is ejected. During relaxation (*diastole*), blood enters the chambers. The atria contract first, propelling their contents into the ventricles. The ventricles, now filled with blood from the period of relaxation and the contraction of the atria, eject their contents, the right ventricle into the lungs and the left ventricle to the rest of the body. For this sequence to occur normally, coordination is needed, and this is supplied by the electrical system of the heart.

Chapter 2

The Heart as an Electrical Organ

In the floor of the right atrium, near the *superior vena cava*, the large vein that collects blood from the upper part of the body, is a structure called the *sinus node*, or *sinoatrial (SA) node*. This collection of cells constitutes the fundamental pacemaker of the heart (Figure 2-1).

The sinus node generates tiny electrical impulses in a regular rhythm, the rate of which is determined by the needs of the body. Fibers from the autonomic nervous system, that part of the nervous system that cannot be voluntarily controlled, modulate the rate that the sinus node discharges. During rest, signals from the vagus nerve, a part of the parasympathetic nervous system, slow the heat rate. During exertion or nervousness, impulses from the vagus nerve decrease, and the sympathetic nervous system and hormones released for this purpose speed the heart and stimulate the chambers to contract more forcefully.

The electrical impulses from the sinus node flow through the muscle and specialized conducting tissue in the two atria causing them to contract. The signal also travels to the *atrioventricular (A-V) node*, another structure in the heart's electrical system, which lies in the floor of the right atrium close to the tricuspid valve and the right ventricle. This collection of specialized cells has an unusual property. It delays

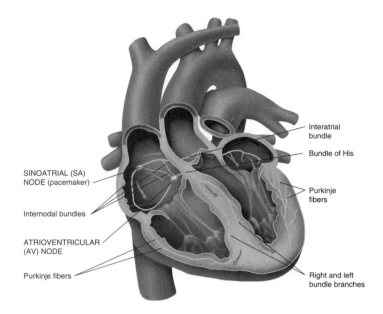

SINOATRIAL (SA)
NODE (pacemaker)

Internodal bundles

ATRIOVENTRICULAR
(AV) NODE

Purkinje fibers

Interatrial
bundle

Bundle of His

Purkinje
fibers

Right and left
bundle branches

FIGURE 2-1   Electrical System of the Heart

transmission of the signal it has received before delivering it to the ventricles. This brief interruption gives the ventricles time to receive the blood the atria are ejecting before contracting and closing the tricuspid and mitral valves. Arrhythmias can occur when this delay is abnormally prolonged or shortened.

After leaving the A-V node, the signal passes through the *bundle of His*, a collection of conducting tissue within the ventricles. From the bundle of His, the signal reaches the *bundle branches* in each of the two ventricles. The right bundle branch consists of a single collection of conducting fibers that travels to the tip or apex of the right ventricle and then spreads within the ventricle activating the ventricular muscle to contract. The left bundle branch quickly ramifies or separates into a wide collection of fibers on the *endocardium*, the internal surface of the left ventricle. These fibers then conduct the electrical signal to the left ventricular muscle and stimulate it to contract in a specific sequence designed to eject the blood most efficiently. The conducting tissues spreading through the ventricles are known as *Purkinje fibers*.

Part II

Patients and Their Arrhythmias

Chapter 3

Premature Beats in a Healthy Student

When I was working as a consultant cardiologist in the student health department of a large university, a 20-year-old undergraduate came to me because, as he said, "My heart is turning over in my chest."

The symptom began with what felt like an early heartbeat followed by a pause and then an unusually strong beat. Although these sequences usually occurred only once, sometimes they seemed to persist with several identical sensations one after the other. I asked him when he was most likely to feel the sensation, and he replied particularly when he was lying in bed waiting to fall asleep and only occasionally during the day. Did he feel lightheaded during the episodes, was his heart beating unusually rapidly, or had he fainted? He answered "no" to each of these questions but did say that when the problem occurred he felt "nervous" and ascribed this to worrying about what the symptom meant. He did not have the sensations each day—only a couple of times each week. Otherwise, he felt well and was able to do everything that he usually did, including playing intramural sports.

I performed a physical examination and found nothing wrong. I then took an electrocardiogram, which was also normal. While the electrocardiogram was running he had none of the sensations.

We call the symptom the patient was experiencing *palpitations*. I could be quite sure that his palpitations were caused by *premature* or early heart-beats, a medical term that, for once, perfectly described what the student was feeling. Premature beats are the most common of the cardiac arrhythmias or abnormalities in the rhythm of the heart that, in most cases, as in the student, can be annoying but not dangerous.

Because the electrocardiogram in the office was unrevealing, I ordered that a small tape recorder be attached to electrodes on the student's skin. I asked him to wear this device for the next 48 hours and to keep a diary of when he had the palpitations. Two days later he delivered the monitor with its cassette tape to my office. We played back the tape, which for the most part showed a normal electrocardiogram. Occasionally, however, single premature beats appeared, and some of these coincided with the times in the diary when the student felt the palpitations, many when he was going to sleep. Many patients with palpitations likely notice them at this time because their minds are then free of other distractions.

The form of the complexes in the electrocardiogram suggested that they originated in the ventricles, the principal pumping chambers of the heart. Premature beats may also start in the atria, the two entry chambers that collect the blood from the body and the lungs and deliver it to the ventricles. The student's history with no limitations in his activities and his normal physical examination and resting electrocardiogram convinced me that, except for the extra beats, his heart was normal. Some doctors might, at this point, order an echocardiogram to evaluate the function of the heart muscle and valves to verify the clinical impression of good health. In view of the anxieties of the student and his family, I had one taken. It was normal.

No drug treatment was indicated for this otherwise healthy young man. I advised him that the premature beats posed no risk to his health, that they might well disappear on their own, and that he should lead a normal life. Accordingly, I encouraged the student to "live with the problem" but to come back to see me if the palpitations continued to bother him.

I never saw him again but heard from my colleagues in the student health department that my advice seemed to have been sufficient. When he returned to student health for another problem, he told the doctor that not only had the number of palpitations decreased but that when he had them they troubled him little because he knew that they were not something that should worry him.

Although our student did not need specific treatment, some people with premature beats but otherwise normal hearts may be so troubled by the symptoms that a drug should be prescribed. Most of us would first turn to one of the beta-adrenergic blocking drugs, which can often reduce or eliminate the premature beats. Other more potent antiarrhythmic drugs are available but are seldom required for this problem.

Chapter 4

Atrial Fibrillation in a Medical Intern

While admitting a patient to the hospital at 3 a.m., a 25-year-old medical intern sensed that his own heart was beating rapidly. Stepping aside from the patient, he took his pulse and counted about 130 beats per minute. He thought that the strength of the beats varied and that the rhythm of the beats was irregular. Although frightened by the experience, he was able to deduce that he was probably in atrial fibrillation. To confirm the diagnosis, the intern went to the emergency department and asked one of his colleagues to take an electrocardiogram. He was in atrial fibrillation—the intern had clearly learned his lessons well—with an average heart rate of about 120 beats per minute. His colleague advised that he be admitted to the hospital, and the intern—exhausted by many hours of work, little sleep, and anxiety because of the diagnosis and the many cups of coffee that he had recently drunk—agreed. Given digoxin, a beta-blocker and a mild sedative, he slept for 8 hours—the most he had slept continuously for several days—and when he awoke, his heart was beating normally.

One of the staff cardiologists then interviewed and examined his doctor/patient. He reported never having had a similar episode in the past and was a vigorous athlete with no limitations on his physical activities. He had never had rheumatic fever or been told of having a heart murmur. The physical examination of his heart was normal, and the electrocardiogram now showed normal rhythm. An echocardiogram, the noninvasive test that best reveals how the cardiac structures are functioning, was normal. Because an overactive thyroid gland can produce atrial fibrillation, blood was drawn to test for hyperthyroidism; the results were normal.

What Is Atrial Fibrillation?

In atrial fibrillation, the atria, the upper, smaller chambers of the heart, do not generate normal electrical impulses and, accordingly, do not contract. This abnormality produces a rapid, irregular beating of the ventricles, the principal pumping chambers of the heart, and this is the symptom that most patients with the arrhythmia sense. Although the most common of the sustained arrhythmias, atrial fibrillation occurs infrequently. For example, in 5,191 adult men and women, chronic atrial fibrillation developed in only 2% during 22 years of study.[*]

American men develop atrial fibrillation as much as 1.5 times as often as women.[†] The greater incidence of coronary heart disease in men probably accounts for much of this difference.[‡] A few cases of atrial fibrillation have been found to occur with familial association. A striking

---

[*] Atrial fibrillation rarely occurs in babies and children or in small animals but does develop in large breeds of dogs and horses. Apparently, the heart, and specifically the atria, must be sufficiently large to sustain the arrhythmia.

[†] "Perhaps because men are generally subject to greater strain than are women," suggested the eminent American cardiologist Paul Dudley White more than 50 years ago[1] (see Chapter 18). Most doctors would not so explain the difference now!

[‡] Do the slightly larger hearts of men when compared with women also influence this incidence?

report, published in 1957,[2] describes the presence of the arrhythmia in five generations of a family. Twenty-one members who lived to the age of 40 developed atrial fibrillation. In the first and second generations, all who lived into or beyond the sixth decade had the arrhythmia.

Although usually associated with intrinsic and often serious heart disease, atrial fibrillation sometimes occurs in people with structurally normal hearts as in our young doctor. The intern had no disease of the myocardium, the muscle that performs the heart's unique function of pumping blood to body, or of the valves of the heart,* which direct the blood in the right direction. The anatomy of his heart showed no evidence of a congenital malformation. His problem was primarily electrical. We call this disease in patients without other types of heart disease *lone* atrial fibrillation, and it occurs in as many as 10% of patients with atrial fibrillation. This does not mean that everything about the heart is normal. Our current methods for evaluating heart disease may be insufficiently precise to detect what is wrong. More than 75% of patients with lone atrial fibrillation are men, for reasons that have never been established. They tend to be younger than is the average for all patients with atrial fibrillation; thus, it is very unlikely that the higher incidence of coronary heart disease in men explains this.

Arterial Pulse

Feeling the pulse in an artery, usually at the wrist, is the principal technique that patients and members of their families employ to recognize atrial fibrillation. An old diagnostic aid of uncertain provenance uses the foot as if it were a metronome. While feeling the pulse, the observer, who may be the patient, starts tapping his foot to what appears to be the rhythm. Because the foot tends to beat regularly, comparison with the pulse can help one recognize the rhythm of atrial fibrillation, which is frequently described as *irregularly irregular* because no consistent pattern can be discerned.

---

* The principal cause of valvular heart disease in the United States used to be rheumatic fever, and for completeness, the cardiologist asked the intern whether he had ever had this disease characterized by arthritis, fever, and cardiac abnormalities. Rheumatic fever occurs so seldom in Americans that many medical students never see a case and overlook the diagnosis if faced with a case. Rheumatic fever and the damage it produces on the heart still plague many patients in some underdeveloped countries.

In atrial fibrillation, the amount of blood entering the ventricles varies with the length of the preceding pause. When the pause is longer, the ventricles fill more completely and vice versa. The more the ventricles fill, the more blood they will eject and the stronger will be the pulse. This accounts for the varying intensity of the pulse when one examines a patient in atrial fibrillation.

When the rate is rapid or the left ventricle diseased, the amount of blood ejected in some of the beats will be small—so small, in some cases, that the observer will feel no pulse even though the left ventricle has contracted. The difference between the rate of the heartbeat and the pulse is known as the *pulse deficit*. The doctor determines this by feeling the pulse and, at the same time, listening to the heart with the stethoscope and noting the number of heartbeats that produce no pulse. Because of the pulse deficit, the therapist must be guided by examining the heartbeat with the stethoscope or from the electrocardiogram, when giving drugs to decrease the heart rate in patients with atrial fibrillation, and not by counting the number of impulses felt in a peripheral vessel. Because the heart rate tends to be somewhat slower and the heart is structurally normal in patients with lone atrial fibrillation, large pulse deficits in patients with this condition are rare.

Lone Atrial Fibrillation Associated with a Slow Heart Rate

In some cases of lone atrial fibrillation, the arrhythmia occurs more often when the patient is resting and the heart rate is slow, either during sleep or after the evening meal. Those whose lone atrial fibrillation starts when the heart rate is slow develop *paroxysms* (episodes) that occur weekly, or more or less frequently, and last from a few minutes to several hours, but seldom permanently. In general, the shorter the paroxysms in these patients, the more frequent the attacks. The cause of this variant appears to be heightened sensitivity of the atria to stimulation from the vagal parasympathetic nervous system, the autonomic* fibers that, among many other functions, slow the heart rate. Drugs that slow the heart rate, like beta-adrenergic blocking drugs, can increase the likelihood that paroxysms will start during the night.

---

* The autonomic nervous system, consisting of the sympathetic and parasympathetic systems, is not under voluntary control.

Treatment

The intern was given digoxin and a beta-blocking drug, both of which decreased the rate of the heart. At the slower rate, the palpitations became less noticeable, and if the intern were active rather than resting, he would have had less fatigue and shortness of breath than before taking the drugs. As sleep restored normal mental and physical function, his heart spontaneously reverted to normal rhythm. This is usually what happens to patients with lone atrial fibrillation, and specific treatment to accomplish this is seldom required.

His cardiologist then reviewed with him what the intern already knew from his studies and had observed during his first episode of the arrhythmia. Many doctors believe that overdosing on stimulants, such as caffeinated beverages and drugs to keep one awake, and long periods of work without sleep predispose patients to recurrences of atrial fibrillation. Alcoholic beverages can also produce episodes in some patients. The intern would try to observe the lessons this information provides.

Further attacks seldom recurred. When they did, he would try to stop working, and after resting, normal rhythm would return. He was able to treat these episodes without being admitted to the hospital. If the arrhythmia had recurred frequently, which they did not, or interfered seriously with his life, an antiarrhythmic drug could be prescribed to suppress the arrhythmia. He began to take low-dose aspirin to protect against a stroke that occurs with increased frequency in patients with atrial fibrillation. This calamity, however, is rare in patients with lone atrial fibrillation who are younger than 60 years of age, and some doctors would not prescribe aspirin for this purpose.

Chapter 5

Atrial Fibrillation in a Man with a Heart Murmur

A 70-year-old accountant came to the emergency department of a community hospital complaining that his heart began beating rapidly and irregularly after finishing dinner 2 hours previously. In addition to the speed and irregularity of the heart, the patient thought that the intensity of the beats varied. An electrocardiogram was taken that confirmed that the rhythm of the heart was irregular and that the average ventricular rate was about 130 beats per minute. The patient had developed atrial fibrillation.

The patient had been in general good health except for hypertension, which had been successfully treated with a beta-blocking drug and lisinopril, an antihypertension drug. He had a heart murmur that was first detected when he was a teenager. When the physician in the emergency department examined him, he heard a systolic murmur* with the characteristics of mitral regurgitation. An echocardiogram confirmed the diagnosis.

---

* Systolic murmurs are heard while the ventricles contract and diastolic murmurs when they relax.

This is the second case of atrial fibrillation described in this book. Medically, however, the patients are quite different. The intern with lone atrial fibrillation described in Chapter 2 was 45 years younger and had no heart disease other than the arrhythmia. This patient has hypertension and mitral regurgitation, both of which can produce atrial fibrillation.

In *mitral regurgitation*—or *mitral insufficiency*, as it is sometimes called—the mitral valve allows blood to leak backward from the left ventricle into the left atrium. The normal mitral valve prevents this from happening and assures that the blood will travel in its normal route from left atrium to left ventricle. The problem is due to an abnormality, possibly congenital and of uncertain cause, that distorts the architecture and function of the valve and its supporting structures and prevents the valve from closing completely when the left ventricle contracts.

Leaking of the mitral valve increases pressure in the left atrium, which will slowly *dilate* (enlarge.) When it dilates sufficiently, and this may take decades, the chamber can no longer sustain the normal, orderly electrical activation of the chamber, and atrial fibrillation may develop. During this arrhythmia, the muscle fibers of the atria twitch rapidly in an uncoordinated manner, no longer in the organized pattern of normal rhythm. The ventricles receive the multiple electrical signals from the fibrillating atria, respond to many of them, and contract rapidly and irregularly.

Causes of Atrial Fibrillation

Our patient had three issues which could contribute to his arrhythmia: age, hypertension, and mitral regurgitation.

Age

Regardless of the type of heart disease, advancing age is the single most important factor encouraging the development of atrial fibrillation in patients with conditions that may produce it, and our patient was now entering his eighth decade.

Hypertension

More patients with hypertension develop atrial fibrillation than those without it. Control of the hypertension should reduce the likelihood of having the arrhythmia.

Valvular Heart Disease

Mitral regurgitation has become a frequent cause of atrial fibrillation in the United States. In the past, disease of the heart's valves caused by rheumatic fever accounted for many cases of atrial fibrillation.

Mitral stenosis (narrowing or constriction) is the principal lesion produced by rheumatic heart disease that most predisposes to atrial fibrillation. In this condition, which is much more likely to occur in women than in men, the amount that the mitral valve opens when blood passes from left atrium to left ventricle gradually decreases because of the inflammation produced by the disease. When this opening becomes sufficiently small, the pressure of the blood in the left atrium increases leading to thickening and enlarging of the chamber. As with mitral regurgitation, the abnormally shaped left atrium interferes with normal electrical function in the atria and produces atrial fibrillation.

Coronary Heart Disease

Most patients with coronary heart disease (also called coronary artery disease) are in normal rhythm. Atrial fibrillation more likely develops in such patients during myocardial infarction, when the development of the arrhythmia reflects rather severe ventricular destruction and predicts a less favorable prognosis than in those with heart attacks who remain in normal rhythm. The incidence of this complication has decreased thanks to contemporary means of treating myocardial infarction in which the occluded coronary artery is opened before the full effects of the obstruction can be produced on the ventricles. The duration of atrial fibrillation during acute myocardial infarction is usually brief. Most patients who develop the arrhythmia and survive the infarction spontaneously return to *sinus* (normal) rhythm.

After Cardiac Surgery

Atrial fibrillation frequently occurs in the early postoperative period after cardiac surgery, including in those patients having the coronary artery bypass graft (CABG) operation. In patients who have not had the arrhythmia previously, postoperative atrial fibrillation is almost always transient, and normal rhythm returns soon either spontaneously or with specific treatment.

Alcohol

Ingestion of alcohol can induce atrial fibrillation. Alcohol-related arrhythmias occur more frequently in younger people, particularly males, than in older patients, where the cause is more likely to be coronary heart disease. Atrial fibrillation can develop during alcohol withdrawal as well as during intoxication.

The association of paroxysmal arrhythmias with weekends and holidays has led to use of the phrase *holiday heart* to characterize such cases. Arrhythmias, including atrial fibrillation, appear to occur both in regular, heavy drinkers and in usually sober individuals who celebrate too emphatically on special occasions. Alcohol-induced atrial fibrillation, of course, is not limited to drinking on weekends or holidays. "After all, ethanol is the culprit instead of Saturdays, Sundays, or holidays," as two investigators have written.[3]

Cardiomyopathy

Atrial fibrillation may complicate the course of patients with *cardiomyopathy*, the disease in which the ventricles contract poorly. Myocardial infarctions and alcohol can produce cardiomyopathy, but in many cases, the cause is unknown. The arrhythmia more likely appears when the disease has become severe and the *ejection fraction*—the frequently used echocardiographic measure of the ability of the left ventricle to contract—is low.

Symptoms of heart failure, such as *dyspnea* (shortness of breath) or *edema* (collection of fluid in the legs and elsewhere), may rapidly worsen when atrial fibrillation develops in patients with severe cardiomyopathy. Atrial fibrillation appearing in patients with the type of cardiomyopathy known as hypertrophic cardiomyopathy can produce particularly troublesome symptoms.

Conversely, when a rapid arrhythmia like atrial fibrillation develops in a patient whose heart is otherwise normal and is not treated, the ventricles may develop a reversible form of cardiomyopathy. In these cases, the ventricles lose normal function and enlarge, producing symptoms of heart failure. Recognition and treatment of the arrhythmia will often re-establish normal function.

Thyrotoxicosis

As many as 25% of patients with an overactive thyroid gland develop atrial fibrillation. This occurs more often in older thyrotoxic patients* and particularly in men possibly because of the presence of concurrent coronary heart disease. Young women with the variant of thyrotoxicosis known as Grave's disease seldom develop atrial fibrillation. Patients without hyperthyroidism who take large doses of thyroid hormone—to try to lose weight, for example—can develop atrial fibrillation.

The likelihood of the intern described in Chapter 2 with lone atrial fibrillation having thyrotoxicosis as the cause of his arrhythmia is very low. Doctors, however, always consider the diagnosis in every patient with atrial fibrillation and order the appropriate blood tests.

Initial Treatment

The patient was given digoxin and additional doses of his beta-blocking drug by intravenous infusion. Within 15 minutes, the rate of the arrhythmia began to slow, which reduced the intensity of the palpitations. He was also given heparin through the intravenous line. The patient was transferred to a cardiac monitoring unit so that the staff could observe his electrocardiogram. The tests for myocardial infarction showed no damage, and the thyroid function was normal.

---

* It was hyperthyroidism that caused the atrial fibrillation that temporarily afflicted former President George H.W. Bush in May, 1991.[4] He developed the arrhythmia while jogging and became short of breath and fatigued. Tests showed that his thyroid was overfunctioning, and this was successfully treated. Subsequently, no further episodes of atrial fibrillation have been reported.

Emboli and Anticoagulation

When the atria fibrillate, the blood no longer flows smoothly from the pulmonary veins of the lung, into the left atrium, past the mitral valve, and into the left ventricle. Some of it, swirling in the left atrium, may form clots that attach themselves to the walls of the left atrium. If these clots are released, they become emboli, which may enter the general circulation and obstruct vessels supplying vital organs such as the brain. The result may be a stroke. Although these calamities are infrequent in patients with atrial fibrillation, they occur more often than in patients in normal rhythm. Anticoagulants such as warfarin (Coumadin), heparin, and aspirin reduce the likelihood that clots will form.

Enough digoxin and beta-blocking drugs were given to maintain an average rate of 70 to 90 beats per minute when the patient was resting. Eighteen hours after developing the arrhythmia, the patient became aware that the palpitations had stopped. The monitor showed that normal rhythm had returned. The patient was discharged on the same medical program plus aspirin. He was instructed to take antibiotics during dental and surgical procedures to prevent infection on his abnormal mitral valve, a serious complication called endocarditis.

This was the patient's first documented episode of atrial fibrillation. He converted to normal rhythm spontaneously possibly assisted by the additional beta-adrenergic blocking drug. The patient continued taking aspirin, which fulfilled two useful roles. For the atrial fibrillation, the drug will provide some protection against clot formation and emboli and will reduce progression of coronary heart disease, for which we have no evidence in this patient at this time.

Warfarin (Coumadin) is the anticoagulant that is most often administered to patients with atrial fibrillation to prevent emboli. It is, however, a drug that can increase bleeding during trauma or some illnesses, and the doctor did not think that this potent agent was needed yet because as far as he and the patient could tell the arrhythmia had occurred only once. (Other physicians might prescribe warfarin at this time.) As for heparin, it can only be given intravenously or by injection, which reduces the convenience of its administration for patients not in the hospital.

More Trouble

The patient had no further episodes of the arrhythmia for almost 2 years. He then recognized that he had developed atrial fibrillation again and came to the doctor's office. After taking an electrocardiogram that confirmed the recurrence of atrial fibrillation, the doctor sent the patient home with instructions to take more beta-adrenergic blocking drug and digoxin until the arrhythmia resolved, which occurred after about 24 hours. While in atrial fibrillation, the patient reported feeling weaker than usual and having shortness of breath while climbing the stairs in his house. The next episode occurred about 1 year later and resolved in 36 hours with the same treatment. After this episode, the doctor prescribed the antiarrhythmic drug amiodarone. He also instructed the patient to take the anticoagulant warfarin to reduce the likelihood that the arrhythmia would produce a stroke. An echocardiogram showed that the mitral regurgitation had worsened and that the left atrium had enlarged further.

The intervals between episodes of paroxysmal atrial fibrillation have decreased, the time needed for conversion has increased, and the symptoms during the arrhythmia have worsened. To reduce the likelihood of further episodes, now quite troublesome to the patient, the doctor prescribed amiodarone, the drug that many cardiologists believe to be the most effective agent to maintain normal rhythm. Concerned about the possibility of emboli, now that the arrhythmia was occurring more often, he advised the patient to take warfarin, the most effective anticoagulant.

The patient now began to notice that his ability to exercise was decreasing and that climbing stairs rapidly produced shortness of breath even when his rhythm was normal. Then, 6 months later, he developed the arrhythmia again associated with shortness of breath while resting, weakness, and anxiety. The doctor admitted him to the hospital.

The patient's blood pressure was 110/80; his usual pressure was 125/75. His skin was slightly sweaty. The doctor could hear the same murmur in his heart and *rales* (crackly sounds) in the lungs. His ankles were edematous with fluid. This abnormal retention of fluid, as shown by the edema and rales, indicated the beginnings of heart failure. To remove the extra fluid, the doctor administered a diuretic, which relieved the dyspnea, and reduced the rales and edema in his legs. Another echocardiogram showed that the mitral regurgitation had worsened, the left atrium had further enlarged, and the contracting ability of the left ventricle had decreased.

By 48 hours, normal rhythm had not returned. The doctor suggested that cardioversion be performed. The patient agreed. This is the treatment familiar to all who watch hospital-based programs on television. Paddles leading from the cardioverter device were placed on the patient's chest. An anesthesiologist administered a short-acting anesthetic so that the patient would not feel the electric shock the cardioverter delivers. When the drug had taken effect, the doctor pressed the button activating the cardioverter. A shock passed through the patient's chest, converting his atrial fibrillation to normal rhythm. After recovering from the anesthetic, the patient said that the arrhythmia was gone. His blood pressure had returned to the value usually present during normal rhythm.

Cardioversion

Despite the amiodarone, the patient's tendency to develop atrial fibrillation had increased. This time, the arrhythmia produced symptoms that were quite troubling to the patient and concerning to his doctor. The sweating and lower blood pressure reflected the body's reaction to the significant reduction in the amount of blood the patient's heart was able to deliver to the body. The dyspnea (shortness of breath) was caused by abnormally high pressure of blood in the lungs, produced as the left ventricle ejected an increasing portion of its blood backward into the left atrium and then into the lungs. These events led to abnormal retention of fluid, some of which had leaked into the lung tissues, producing the rales the doctor heard and contributing to the patient's dyspnea. Normal atrial contraction had now become essential to sustain normal cardiac function, and when it disappeared during atrial fibrillation, severe symptoms resulted.

Although the patient and his doctor might have waited longer for spontaneous reversion to normal rhythm to occur, the symptoms bothered the patient and worried his physician enough that the doctor turned to the most definitive way of suppressing the arrhythmia. Synchronized cardioversion, in which the shock is delivered at the time during the heart's cycle in which the fewest complications are likely to occur, is almost always effective in converting intermittent atrial fibrillation. The same cannot be said for many patients with permanent atrial fibrillation for whom the treatment may be ineffective.

Transesophageal Echocardiogram

In some cases, a transesophageal echocardiogram is performed before the cardioversion to determine whether a clot is present in the left atrium, which the shock of the conversion might dislodge and produce a stroke. For this procedure, the patient is given a sedative, and a tube is passed through the mouth into his esophagus, much as a gastroenterologist performs endoscopy of the upper esophagus, stomach, and small intestine. In this case, however, rather than a lens at the tip of the tube, there is a transistor that transmits and detects sound waves directed where the operator specifies. Part of the esophagus lies close to the left atrium, and its size and contents can be clearly seen with this technique. If clots are found, the cardioversion is postponed, unless required in an emergency, and the patient is given anticoagulants for at least 3 weeks.

Our patient did not receive a transesophageal echocardiogram because he was taking the anticoagulant drug Coumadin in sufficient amounts to produce the full therapeutic effect of the drug and prevent the formation of clots in the left atrium. If, however, he had not been taking such a drug or if the dose had been inadequate, the doctor would obtain a transesophageal echocardiogram.

Surgery

The doctor told the patient that in all likelihood the frequency of episodes of atrial fibrillation would increase and that the symptoms during paroxysms would worsen. The leaky mitral valve was the culprit, enlarging the left atrium, perpetuating the arrhythmia, and reducing the heart's output even during normal rhythm. To characterize the malfunction of the mitral valve, the cardiologist performed a transesophageal echocardiogram, which showed that the regurgitation had now become severe and that both leaflets of the valve were involved. A cardiac surgeon was consulted who agreed that the valve should be repaired, and the patient consented to the operation. Cardiac catheterization was performed to determine whether the patient also had significant coronary disease. He did not.

The operation was performed 2 days later, and the surgeon was able to repair the valve so that little leaking remained. To prevent further episodes of atrial fibrillation, he ablated specific areas in the atria with radiofrequency current. This procedure interrupts the circuits sustaining the atrial fibrillation and, in most cases, prevents the arrhythmia from recurring.

The patient's postoperative course was uneventful. For several months, he continued to take amiodarone and warfarin. One year later, the patient remained in normal rhythm, and his exercise ability had returned to its normal level. The amiodarone and anticoagulation were discontinued.

The intensity of the symptoms that patients develop when they have atrial fibrillation varies greatly. Some barely notice them; others are disabled by them. Our patient's symptoms increased as mitral regurgitation, the cause of the arrhythmia in his case, worsened. If the valve had not been repaired or replaced with a prosthesis if repair was not possible, it is likely that the episodes of paroxysmal atrial fibrillation would have occurred more frequently, that cardioversion would have been required to restore sinus rhythm, and that eventually, the arrhythmia would have been present most of the time.

Catheter Ablation

This technique, the cardiologist's answer to surgical ablation, as performed on our patient, is now being applied for the treatment of paroxysmal atrial fibrillation in the electrophysiology laboratory.

Many episodes of paroxysmal atrial fibrillation begin with premature beats originating in the pulmonary veins. If these sites can be electrically separated from the atria, the arrhythmia may be prevented. Using an electrode catheter, the electrophysiologist burns tracks into the portion of the left atrium that encircle the pulmonary veins, thereby preventing the premature beats from activating the atria and producing atrial fibrillation. At this time (2005), the procedure is effective in ridding the patient of the arrhythmia in about 75% of cases.

Chapter 6

Supraventricular Tachycardia (SVT) in a Healthy Young Woman

A 25-year-old editor consulted me because of palpitations that she had had for several months. She would be reading or watching television when suddenly and without warning she felt her heart racing. She took her pulse and timed it at about 140 beats per minute. She thought the rhythm was regular.

The patient is experiencing one of the *tachyarrhythmias* (rapid cardiac rhythm disturbances). Can we deduce from the history alone which one it is? Let us start with lone atrial fibrillation as discussed in Chapter 1. Our medical intern felt that his pulse was irregular, whereas this patient sensed regularity. This is a helpful observation although not foolproof, since the faster the heart rate, the greater difficulty one has in deciding whether the pulse is regular or irregular. If she is correct, we can eliminate atrial fibrillation.

I asked her to simulate the rate and rhythm of the tachycardia by tapping with her finger. This trick can sometimes help define what is going on, and in this case, the tapping did seem regular and rapid.

We should next consider *sinus tachycardia*, the normal rapid heart rhythm produced by exertion or anxiety. In this case, the patient was resting when the rapid heart action began. Our patient believed that the arrhythmia began and ended suddenly without any unusual sensation preceding it. Sinus tachycardia tends to develop and terminate relatively gradually. Let us hear some of her other observations.

> When the tachycardia began, she became weak and lightheaded when standing and, thinking she might faint, would often sit or lie down. Fatigue and shortness of breath made climbing stairs difficult, which was never the case in normal rhythm. The intensity of these symptoms, worse when the tachycardia began, characteristically lessened in the next few minutes.

These symptoms suggest that the amount of blood the heart ejects per minute has significantly decreased. When standing, she cannot sustain blood flow and blood pressure adequate to provide normal perfusion of the brain—producing the light-headedness—or the body—causing fatigue and breathlessness. Reduced perfusion of the lungs and increased blood pressure within the lungs produce her dyspnea on exertion.

That she began to feel somewhat better after a few minutes reflects the body's accommodating to the abnormal condition by rallying neurological and endocrinological forces that partially counter the lowering effects of the tachycardia on the blood pressure.

> Sometimes she would feel a burning sensation in the front of her chest.

This is a symptom many patients with this form of tachycardia observe. It may sound somewhat like *angina pectoris*, the chest pressure patients with coronary heart disease feel when they exert themselves and the heart receives an inadequate supply of blood because of the obstructions in the coronary arteries. However, in a young person such as our patient, coronary disease is extremely unlikely. We do not fully understand what produces the chest pain in these cases.

The arrhythmia and the associated symptoms, which could last for a few seconds or as long as 30 minutes, would stop suddenly and unexpectedly. Sometimes, she discovered, coughing seemed to terminate the arrhythmia. She also reported having to pass large amounts of urine during some of her more prolonged attacks. She thought that some members of her family might have the same problem but was not sure.

Just as the arrhythmia started, it stopped—suddenly and without warning. This is not characteristic of sinus tachycardia, which gradually slows as the cause for the rapid beating passes. Coughing is one of maneuvers that patients either discover or are instructed about that can terminate such arrhythmias by activating the autonomic nervous system, those fibers not under voluntary control.

As for the *polyuria* (much urine), this commonly accompanies several of the tachyarrhythmias. As of 2005, we have not proven why this occurs although several theories have been proposed.

I found nothing wrong when I examined her heart. Her electrocardiogram was also normal.

This was expected. Most young patients with these arrhythmias have normal hearts except for the electrical structures that sustain the tachycardia. Their heart muscle, valves, and coronary arteries are normal. Accordingly, the electrocardiogram is characteristically normal except in the Wolff-Parkinson-White syndrome, which is discussed later.

I then gave her a device that would record her electrocardiogram when she activated it during an episode of tachycardia and told her to return after the next episode. If paroxysms of tachycardia recurred, I suggested she try bearing down as if she were trying to move her bowels, that this technique, called the Valsalva maneuver, might convert the arrhythmia. The patient returned 3 weeks later. She had had an episode of tachycardia on the previous day that she terminated by performing the Valsalva maneuver. She had activated the recorder during the tachycardia. Analysis of the record showed that the heart rate was 180 beats per minute, that the rhythm was regular, and that the tachycardia had begun and ended suddenly.

History of Patients with Supraventricular Tachycardia

This patient's story about her arrhythmia is what one usually hears from patients with this problem. The first episodes of supraventricular tachycardia (SVT) tend to occur between the ages of 15 and 35 years—she was 25 years old—although a few experience their first paroxysms at about the age of 50 years. Among children, the first episode occurs most often from birth to 2 months of age, and next most frequently from ages 5 to 10 years. Fetuses, premature newborns, and infants may develop SVT.

Probably as many men as women develop SVT, although the sex distribution is slightly different depending on the mechanism of the arrhythmia. Cardiac disease in addition to the arrhythmia is more likely to be present in men than in women with SVT.

Patients can frequently recall events in their lives that seem to precipitate, or be associated with, episodes such as a certain body movement, an emotional upset, or a dream. Some episodes seem to occur at specific times during the menstrual cycle. Patients occasionally sustain their first episode of SVT during pregnancy, but the arrhythmia need not interfere with the normal course of pregnancy even though some women report that pregnancy seems to increase the number of paroxysms.

The frequency with which paroxysms recur and the duration of a single attack may vary from patient to patient from many attacks per day to only an occasional one per year, but they tend to maintain a particular pattern in the individual case. The more often arrhythmias occurred in the past, the more likely will they recur in the future.

Predicting when a paroxysm will appear, however, is almost impossible. Thus, in general, the time of a previous episode does not forecast when the next episode will occur.

Symptoms Produced by SVT

SVT lasting for at least 30 seconds produces symptoms that few patients can ignore. As with our patient, most decrease their activity during an attack, and many find it necessary to sit or lie down. A few, however, are unaware when having a paroxysm. Observers may detect the tachycardia in patients unaware of their own rapid heart action, as described in 1971:[5]

> Cigarettes in a shirt pocket moving in time to the heartbeat, or, as noted by the wife of a patient, movement of the bed in time to the rate of the heart.

Although palpitations are a frequent, although not universal, complaint of patients with SVT, they do not always indicate a clinical arrhythmia. For example, more than two thirds of patients whose SVT has been cured by the procedure known as ablation report the persistence of symptoms similar to those before the arrhythmia was treated.

Many patients with SVT report the sensation of rapid, regular pounding in the neck. This is due to the simultaneous contraction of the right atrium and right ventricle, an abnormal state, which forces blood back into the veins of the neck and body with each beat.

I have described the chest pain our patient developed.

Few patients with SVT faint from the arrhythmia, although many, like our patient become lightheaded or dizzy. Among those who do faint, older patients predominate. SVT rarely causes cardiac arrest.

Our patient confirmed that her paroxysms of SVT started suddenly and ended abruptly, a characteristic feature of SVT. The symptoms that the tachycardia produces may simulate panic, anxiety, or stress. Occasionally, the condition is misdiagnosed as due to one of these common problems.

Treatment—Physical Actions

I instructed our patient in the use of the Valsalva maneuver, one of a group of physical actions that may convert SVT. She had already discovered that coughing seemed to produce normal rhythm.

Some of the maneuvers that patients frequently employ are:

- *Assuming the dependent position* with the head below the rest of the body or leaning over with the head down especially from the squatting or sitting position. Some patients know this maneuver while squatting as hunkering down.
- *Sighing or deep respirations*
- *Coughing*
- *Gagging*
- *Valsalva maneuver*, bearing down as if moving one's bowels, which is more effective when the patient is lying down than standing

The following should usually be performed only by a trained person attending the patient:

- *Carotid sinus massage* in which the operator partially compresses and strokes one of the carotid arteries in the neck, which activates a neurological circuit sometimes converting the arrhythmia
- *Eyeball pressure*
- *Insertion of a nasogastric tube*, which is seldom employed because of the discomfort produced by it
- *Diving reflex* activated by immersing the patient's face in cold water. Energetic patients can perform this maneuver themselves to convert their arrhythmia and the maneuver seems to be particularly effective in infants

These maneuvers seem to be more effective in younger patients. Taking drugs that block the autonomic nervous system such as beta-blockers inhibits the action of these maneuvers in converting the arrhythmia.

Treatment—Drugs

A few weeks later, the patient sustained a particularly troublesome episode. Despite trying all of the maneuvers I had suggested, the arrhythmia continued. Feeling increasingly weak and worried, she called an ambulance and came to the emergency department of the hospital where I worked. She told the staff and me that she was quite uncomfortable, distressed by the palpitations produced by the tachycardia and weak, slightly lightheaded, and short of breath. The symptoms had never previously disabled her so much.

Her blood pressure was 90/70, the systolic (first) pressure significantly below her normal level of 115. Her skin was cool and slightly sweaty. The electrocardiogram confirmed that she was in SVT at a rate of 170 beats per minute. We tried another Valsalva maneuver, and I administered carotid sinus massage, both to no avail. It was time to give a drug that would convert the arrhythmia. An intravenous line was started, and I administered adenosine. Within seconds, normal rhythm returned. She immediately felt much better.

When physical maneuvers do not work and the tachycardia has not spontaneously converted within a reasonable period of time, the patient should seek medical attention in a doctor's office or hospital emergency department. Alternatively, appropriately trained personnel of some ambulances and mobile coronary care units can sometimes carry out the conversion in the patient's home.

For quick conversion of the arrhythmia, most doctors give intravenous doses of adenosine, diltiazem, or verapamil.

Adenosine, probably the most frequently used drug for acute treatment, converts most paroxysms of SVT in adults and children. After doses of 6 and 12 milligrams given sequentially, as required, SVT usually terminates. The most commonly encountered side effects are facial flushing, shortness of breath, and chest pain or pressure. Adenosine slows the normal rhythm of the heart, and this may be seen for a while after conversion. Any side effects that occur persist for only a short time.

Diltiazem and its relative *verapamil*, given intravenously like adenosine, convert most patients to normal rhythm. The side effects are similar among all three except that they last longer with diltiazem and verapamil than those produced by adenosine whose biological effect is quickly dissipated. Diltiazem and verapamil are seldom used today, having been superseded by adenosine.

Other drugs with antiarrhythmic action that convert SVT include amiodarone, beta-adrenergic blocking drugs, and digitalis—the mainstay for this purpose decades ago. It is seldom necessary to use these or one of the several others. They tend to be less effective, slower acting, or cause more side effects than adenosine, diltiazem, or verapamil.

Cardioversion with an externally administered shock will convert almost all cases of SVT; however, one seldom has to use it because drugs are usually effective.

The patient asked what could be done to prevent such attacks in the future. She worried that she might have more frequent, severe attacks and whether the illness was potentially fatal. I assured her that we have several effective methods of preventing further attacks or lessening their intensity if they should recur and that almost no one with SVT dies of it.

I told her that we had two general approaches to treatment at this time: taking a drug that might prevent or lessen the intensity of the attacks or ablating the pathway in the heart supporting the arrhythmia. After hearing about what ablation entails, she elected to try drugs, a very reasonable approach. I prescribed 120 milligrams of diltiazem (Cardizem) per day.

Although she did not have any episodes as disabling as the one that brought her to the hospital, further paroxysms of SVT recurred, and the frequency was not reduced when the dose of diltiazem was increased. We discussed what to do next. I suggested we could try another antiarrhythmic drug, such as a beta-blocker or amiodarone, which might be more effective. I also emphasized that SVT in some patients spontaneously disappears, although it is difficult to predict when and in whom this will happen. In such cases, perpetual treatment is not required, and patients may reasonably try stopping drugs when paroxysms cease. This uncertain future, however, did not particularly appeal to her, and she asked me to tell her about ablation.

Treatment—Ablation

Ablation interrupts the circuit sustaining the tachycardia. It is done as part of an electrophysiological study. By recording from signals detected in the heart, the electrophysiologist locates the circuit that sustains the arrhythmia. He or she then passes radiofrequency current into the pathway, thereby destroying, *ablating*, its ability to conduct electrical activity. With the circuit no longer able to operate, the circuit sustaining the tachycardia can no longer function. When the treatment is effective, and it is in over 90% of cases, the patient is cured of the arrhythmia.

The electrophysiological study is safe and only occasionally produces complications. One of them is the production of heart block—which is very uncommon (see Chapter 9)—requiring the insertion of a pacemaker.

Our patient spent about 3 hours in the electrophysiology laboratory. She was given light sedation to relieve the anxiety experienced by most patients undergoing such a study, but except when a local anesthetic was administered where the electrode catheters were inserted, she felt no pain. She did, however, have several bouts of her typical tachycardia early in the study caused by electrical stimulation of her atria and ventricles used to study the electrophysiologic characteristics of her tachycardia. The electrophysiologist determined that the circuit sustaining the arrhythmia was in the atrioventricular node, the structure on the floor of the right atrium that participates in the transmission of electrical impulses from atria to ventricles. After ablation of part of the circuit sustaining the arrhythmia, stimulation no longer started the arrhythmia, showing that the tachycardia-sustaining circuit had been successfully interrupted.

After making sure that bleeding from the sites where the catheters were introduced had stopped and that the patient had recovered from the sedation, the doctor discharged her several hours later on the same day that the procedure was performed. The patient has had no further episodes of tachycardia.

Wolff-Parkinson-White (WPW) Syndrome

Patients with the Wolff-Parkinson-White syndrome have extra conducting tissue, called accessory pathways, that connect the atria and ventricles and provide an electrophysiological conduit that sustains SVT. One recognizes that the patient has the Wolff-Parkinson-White syndrome from the electrocardiogram, which contains clues to the presence of an abnormal pathway.

Treatment of the SVT that occurs in patients with the Wolff-Parkinson-White syndrome is analogous to the treatment of our patient with SVT sustained in the A-V node. Similar drugs and ablation are effective. During ablation to cure SVT in patients with the Wolff-Parkinson-White syndrome, the electrophysiologist burns the accessory pathway rather than a pathway in the A-V node as in patients with SVT sustained in that structure.

The Wolff-Parkinson-White syndrome is named for Drs. Louis Wolff, John Parkinson, and Paul Dudley White who first described patients with the condition in 1930 (see Chapter 18).

Chapter 7

Atrial Flutter in a 45-Year-Old Executive

A 45-year-old executive for a pharmaceutical company was referred to me because of atrial flutter that amiodarone was not controlling. Two years previously, he was suddenly aware that his heart was beating very rapidly and that he was somewhat short of breath. Because the pulse was so fast, he could not be sure of the rate, but he thought that the rhythm was regular. He went to a hospital where the electrocardiogram showed atrial flutter with a ventricular rate of 150 per minute.

In atrial flutter, electrical impulses circle through abnormal pathways of cardiac tissue in the right atrium at rates of between 250 and 350 per minute. Because the atrioventricular node cannot transmit so many atrial signals, the ventricular rate is a fraction, usually half, of the atrial flutter rate. Even so, the ventricular rate is quite rapid, 150 per minute being typical. If one ventricular beat is produced from each two flutter beats, the ventricular rhythm will be regular, as is the atrial rhythm.

The symptoms during flutter are similar to those patients experience during atrial fibrillation: palpitations—probably the most frequent symptom of all—perception of rapid heart action, dyspnea and breath-lessness, weakness and light-headedness, and what two distinguished British cardiologists from a previous generation called "disinclination for effort."[6] Chest pain occasionally occurs that may or may not indicate the presence of coronary heart disease. Few patients with flutter faint. Symptoms are more disturbing when the ventricular rate is rapid, when the arrhythmia is paroxysmal rather than chronic, and when heart disease is advanced.

> The patient was offered cardioversion, which he accepted. After giving him a short-acting anesthetic, the doctor administered one external shock, which restored the patient to sinus (normal) rhythm.

Cardioversion almost always converts atrial flutter to sinus rhythm as it did in this case.

Causes of Atrial Flutter

> An echocardiogram showed no abnormalities of the heart's muscle or valves. The size of each chamber was normal.

This patient has what we may call *lone* atrial flutter. Lone means that, as far as our tests can tell, his heart is normal except for the arrhythmia. Although we formerly thought that most patients with flutter had heart disease in addition to the arrhythmia, recent studies have shown that as many as half of patients with atrial flutter have none, or to be precise, no heart disease which we can detect.

Those patients with flutter and intrinsic heart disease are most likely to have coronary heart disease or hypertension. This is reasonable because these two problems are the most common cardiovascular diseases in the United States. Flutter, however, unlike atrial fibrillation, rarely complicates the course of patients during or immediately after myocardial infarction.

Lung disease is a relatively common cause of atrial flutter. Intoxication with alcohol produces atrial flutter but only about half as often as it produces atrial fibrillation (*holiday heart syndrome*).

The arrhythmia also appears temporarily after cardiac surgery although infrequently after operations on other parts of the body. Certain congenital defects are associated with flutter, which may also appear after operations to correct congenital abnormalities in the atria. Atrial flutter develops occasionally in patients with cardiomyopathy and *chronic constrictive pericarditis*, in which the sac surrounding the heart has become thickened and restricts the normal motion of the heart.

Treatment

During the next 2 years, the patient had three episodes of atrial flutter. After the second one, his doctor gave him the antiarrhythmic drug amiodarone and the anticoagulant warfarin (Coumadin), but when the arrhythmia recurred 4 months later, he referred the patient to me for possible ablative treatment.

Atrial flutter, as in this case, can be a troublesome arrhythmia to treat. The British cardiologist Paul Wood called it "a relatively uncommon but capricious rhythm, and may occur when least expected," and Albert Waldo of Case Western Reserve University medical school, who has studied the arrhythmia throughout his career, describes it as "a nuisance arrhythmia."[7]

Before ablation and the more effective antiarrhythmic drugs became available, suppressing flutter often required large doses of the drugs then available, which produced troublesome side effects. In many patients, the arrhythmia could not be suppressed, and we administered drugs like digitalis and, more recently, beta-blocking drugs, which reduced symptoms by decreasing the ventricular rate through limiting the number of atrial impulses which could reach the ventricles.

Like atrial fibrillation, atrial flutter predisposes the patient to thromboembolic episodes in which small blood clots can leave the heart and occlude important arteries producing, occasionally, disabling strokes. Consequently, most cardiologists prescribe an anticoagulant to reduce the likelihood of this occurring.

With ablation of the circuit sustaining atrial flutter, we can now offer a definitive cure in most cases. As far as the patient is concerned, the procedure of ablation for flutter is the same as that for SVT described in Chapter 6. The principal difference is that the electrophysiologist works on the circuit sustaining the arrhythmia in the right atrium rather than within the A-V node or an accessory pathway as in patients with SVT. After locating the appropriate place, he or she burns the tissue of the pathway with radiofrequency current. Measurements taken on the residual electrical activity in this area will indicate whether the circuit has been adequately obliterated. If not, additional burns will be administered. As with this form of treatment for SVT, the ablation itself is painless.

The patient was discharged on the day after the ablation. His amiodarone was stopped, and during the next 2 years, he had no more episodes of atrial flutter. With the arrhythmia suppressed, the anticoagulant was also discontinued.

Chapter 8

Multifocal Atrial Tachycardia in a 75-Year-Old Housewife with Emphysema and Diabetes

While being treated in the hospital intensive care unit for an exacerbation of emphysema, this patient's heart rate suddenly increased to a rate of 130 beats per minute. Although short of breath from her lung disease, she did not think that it had recently become worse. Her blood pressure dropped from 140/80 to 120/70, and her temperature was 101°F. When called to see this patient, I found her to be somewhat short of breath sitting in bed, but the staff told me this was no worse than before the tachycardia was noticed. An electrocardiogram had been taken that showed that the rhythm was irregular. The tracing also indicated that the arrhythmia seemed to be originating from several different places in the atrium rather than solely from its normal site in the sinus note.

This is a sick woman. In addition to her lung disease and now the arrhythmia, she also has diabetes, for which she needs insulin, and 4 years ago, she had a myocardial infarction of moderate severity. Before she came into the hospital, she could walk only a few city blocks before having to stop because of shortness of breath. She and her husband live in a retirement home with no steps to climb and eat most of their meals in the facility's restaurant. Twice before, when her dyspnea had worsened, she was admitted to the hospital for treatment of her lung disease. So far, I had detected no evidence of heart failure, and as far as I knew, her heart rhythm had been normal until now.

The arrhythmia that the patient now had is called *multifocal atrial tachycardia*, a name in which each word describes what is going on. It is a tachycardia that is multifocal, originating in several places in the atria. It was recognized as an arrhythmia distinct from atrial fibrillation and other entities as recently as the late 1960s.[8]

The patients it affects have a clinical picture that is familiar to doctors who take care of patients with lung and heart disease or staff intensive care units. They tend to be older; many have lung disease, and some have diabetes. Heart disease is also frequently present, which is not unexpected in view of the age of most patients with the arrhythmia. Multifocal atrial tachycardia also appears in patients after major surgery, particularly when recovery is complicated by pneumonia, infections, or congestive heart failure. For reasons not understood, it seldom occurs during myocardial infarction.

Her pulmonologist, with whom I had cared for several patients with multifocal atrial tachycardia in the past, then joined me, and we discussed what to do. She suspected that the fever was due to bronchitis, which should respond to appropriate antibiotics, and these had been given when the patient was admitted on the previous day.

My colleague then reminded me that several of the drugs used to treat her lung disease could aggravate the arrhythmia, and thus, to the extent possible, the amounts of those being administered were reduced. The staff in the unit energetically assisted her breathing with a ventilator and removed secretions that were collecting in her lungs. She was given an appropriate amount of supplementary oxygen.

What could I as a cardiologist do to help? First, I tried to determine whether she was in congestive heart failure. This is difficult to do in a patient with severe lung disease. The lungs were full of the abnormal sounds produced by the emphysema and bronchitis, masking the sounds that I was trying to hear as evidence of fluid in her lungs. An X-ray, however, suggested the presence of edema in her lungs, and I ordered that she receive a diuretic. I also decided to administer digitalis to improve the function of her heart, whose ability to eject blood was abnormal from the old myocardial infarction and might now be further depressed by her acute illness. Despite her difficulties, the heart rate did not exceed 120 beats per minute most of the time; she had no chest pain, and the electrocardiogram showed no signs of *ischemia* (insufficient blood supply to the heart muscle).

During the next 48 hours, her lung function improved, her fever disappeared, and coincident with the improvement in her pulmonary disease, the multifocal atrial tachycardia disappeared and sinus rhythm returned.

Unlike with most arrhythmias where we concentrate on restoring normal rhythm with drugs or electrical conversion, with multifocal atrial tachycardia, we concentrate on alleviating the underlying, usually acute, illnesses that have produced the arrhythmia. In our patient's case, this involved improving her lung function as quickly as possible and, to some extent, relieving the effects of the acute illness on her heart. In addition, the staff in the intensive care unit concentrated on keeping her diabetes under tight control and fixing any metabolic abnormalities of elements such as potassium and magnesium.

Treating multifocal atrial tachycardia begins by improving the underlying diseases the patient has, in this case, cardiac, pulmonary, metabolic, and infectious conditions that have given rise to the arrhythmia. Frequently, multifocal atrial tachycardia will resolve after such measures without specific antiarrhythmic therapy. Multifocal atrial tachycardia, however, frequently recurs during exacerbations of the underlying diseases.

Chapter 9

Ventricular Tachycardia in a Man with Coronary Heart Disease

I met this 65-year-old, retired grocery store owner when he came to the emergency department of the hospital where I was working. He was complaining of a rapid heartbeat, lightheadedness, and shortness of breath. He was sweaty, obviously short of breath, and frightened. His blood pressure was only 90/70, and his heart rate was 150 beats per minute. The electrocardiogram showed that he was in ventricular tachycardia.

Ventricular tachycardia is a dangerous arrhythmia that originates in diseased ventricles and occasionally in otherwise healthy ventricles. The rapid rate of this abnormal rhythm in a sick heart produces the symptoms my patient felt. He might also have fainted or had chest pain. Unless medical treatment is administered quickly, a patient with ventricular tachycardia may die.

After the diagnosis had been established, the patient was prepared for cardioversion. Paddles leading from the cardioverter device were placed on the patient's chest. An anesthesiologist administered a short-acting drug so that the patient would not feel the electric shock the cardioverter delivers. When the drug had taken effect, I pressed the button activating the cardioverter. A shock passed through the patient's chest, converting his ventricular tachycardia to normal rhythm. When he awoke, he was aware that his heart was no longer beating abnormally and that his shortness of breath was gone. The blood pressure had risen to a normal 130/80, and his heart rate was 85 beats per minute.

After he was fully awake, he told us that he had had a heart attack (myocardial infarction) 3 years previously from which he recovered without complications. Since then, he had been taking aspirin, metoprolol (a beta-adrenergic blocking drug), and simvastatin to lower his low-density lipoprotein cholesterol.

The cause of ventricular tachycardia in most adult patients is chronic coronary heart disease, and this patient was no exception, having had a myocardial infarction in the past. Because most patients with ventricular tachycardia will have further episodes, effective treatment must be administered since sooner or later the arrhythmia will be fatal. Until recently, we prescribed antiarrhythmic drugs to prevent ventricular tachycardia, but these drugs are often ineffective. Fortunately, for the past 2 decades, we have the implantable cardioverter defibrillator, which will convert ventricular tachycardia automatically.

Implantable Cardioverter-Defibrillator

Before inserting the device, most cardiologists want to know the status of the coronary arteries of a patient with a history of coronary heart disease—the previous myocardial infarction proves that he has the disease. In this case, we performed an exercise test that showed no evidence of inadequate blood flow to the heart during physical stress, a condition that we call *ischemia*. Some doctors might want to see the results of cardiac catheterization before inserting a defibrillator, but in the absence of any symptoms suggesting ischemia—the classic one is chest pain on exertion—we concluded that the exercise test constituted an adequate evaluation and, with the patient's permission, proceeded with the operation.

Implantable cardioverter-defibrillators are inserted in the electrophysiology laboratory, an operating room filled with computerized electronic equipment. The device consists of electrodes that convey the therapeutic charge to the ventricles, and a generator, which produces the shock (Figure 14-2 on page 91). The device constantly monitors the cardiac rhythm through the electrical impulses produced by the heart muscle. These tiny signals travel through the electrodes to the generator where a miniature computer evaluates their significance according to instructions that the doctor has programmed into the unit.

My patient was brought to the electrophysiology laboratory and transferred to the operating table. Adhesive patches were attached to his skin. These were connected to wires that led to monitors that record the electrical activity of the heart and through which shocks can be delivered as required. The electrophysiologist administered a local anesthetic into the upper chest wall, made an incision there, and located one of the large veins in this area. Through this vein he then threaded the electrodes into the heart. Satisfied that the electrodes were in the proper location, he attached them to the generator. The electrophysiologist next tested the device to be sure that it would do what it was designed to do.

This requires producing the arrhythmia and then allowing the cardioverter defibrillator to convert it. The electrophysiologist induces the arrhythmia by pacing the ventricle. With the arrhythmia now present in the controlled environment of the electrophysiology laboratory, the generator automatically produces normal rhythm by one or both of two methods: pacing or cardioversion.

The electrophysiologist programs the generator to produce rapid pacing impulses whenever it detects the arrhythmia. Because the amplitude of the impulses produced during pacing is so small, the patient does not feel them, although he or she may be aware when his or her arrhythmia starts a few seconds before the pacing begins. Pacing in the laboratory usually stops ventricular tachycardia and would do so if the arrhythmia recurred at home.

Pacing does not always work, however, and when this happens, the generator discharges a cardioverting shock, which almost always produces normal rhythm. Unfortunately, the converting shock can be felt. Patients describe it as a sudden, although short-lived, pressure and pain within the chest. Because these shocks must be tested during the electrophysiological study, patients are given a short-acting sedative to reduce awareness of the shocks that the generator produces during the study.

Satisfied that the instrument was operating properly, the electrophysiologist closed the incision in the chest wall and applied a bandage. I discharged the patient a day later. He returned in 6 months and reported that he had had no episodes of arrhythmia. However, when we electronically asked the generator what had happened—a process known as *interrogation*—we saw that he had had a few episodes of ventricular tachycardia and that the device had quickly paced him into normal rhythm. As the patient observed, the implantable cardioverter defibrillator had not shocked. The instrument was functioning as designed.

Fortunately, the device controlled the patient's arrhythmia. If the patient had continued to have more frequent episodes, some requiring shocks, I might have given him the antiarrhythmic drug amiodarone, which can suppress paroxysms of ventricular tachycardia. Although helpful in treating the arrhythmia, amiodarone is not always effective, and thus, patients with ventricular tachycardia, whether or not they are taking the drug, need the protection of an implantable cardioverter defibrillator. Electrophysiologists may also try to ablate the circuits in the patient's ventricle that sustains the arrhythmia, a technique that has recently been refined to suppress ventricular tachycardia in many patients.

Thumpversion

Devotees of medical programs on television may have seen a doctor strike her patient's chest with his fist. This action, the first step in the resuscitation of some patients with a potentially fatal ventricular arrhythmia, may restore sinus rhythm in patients with ventricular tachycardia. *Thumpversion* generates a small electrical current in the heart that can interrupt the mechanism that sustains the arrhythmia. Usually, however, this maneuver is unsuccessful, and cardioversion is required.

Chapter 10

Ventricular Fibrillation Producing Cardiac Arrest

While being examined by his doctor because of chest pain during exertion, a 55-year-old laborer suddenly lost consciousness. His doctor felt no pulse and began administering closed chest massage as the nurse prepared the external defibrillator. When the paddles were placed on the patient's chest, the recorder showed ventricular fibrillation. A shock was administered, normal rhythm returned, and the patient regained consciousness. He was admitted to the coronary care unit at a nearby hospital where studies showed he had had a myocardial infarction. When asked about what occurred in the doctor's office, he remembered having chest pain and then becoming lightheaded and weak just before passing out.

In ventricular fibrillation, the orderly process of contraction in the ventricles is replaced by diffuse twitching of the cardiac muscle fibers, which causes the ventricles to stop ejecting blood. Of all of the body's organs, the brain can least tolerate loss of blood flow. Within seconds, the centers controlling consciousness malfunction, and the patient faints. Unless normal heart function quickly returns, brain tissue controlling other vital functions begins to fail, other organs stop working normally from lack of blood, and within minutes, the patient dies. If someone takes the pulse or listens to the heart during ventricular fibrillation, he or she will feel no pulse and hear no heart sounds.

Ventricular fibrillation, or a form of ventricular tachycardia called multiform ventricular tachycardia, is the most serious arrhythmia that complicates myocardial infarction. Ventricular fibrillation rarely reverts spontaneously to normal rhythm. More frequently, the arrhythmia continues until either the arrhythmia is converted by electric shock administered by an implantable cardioverter defibrillator, if the patient has one, or by external cardioversion as in our case. Without this treatment given soon after the arrhythmia develops, the patient will die.

In the coronary care unit, the monitor of his electrocardiogram displayed short bursts of ventricular tachycardia and frequent ventricular premature beats. An echocardiogram showed that the infarction had severely depressed the ability of his left ventricle to contract. His ejection fraction, a measurement the ability of the left ventricle to eject blood, was less than 30%. The normal left ventricular ejection fraction is 55% or greater. His doctors advised that he receive an implantable cardioverter defibrillator, and the patient agreed.

Most patients with myocardial infarction and all with dangerous arrhythmias are admitted to coronary care units, a most important facility first developed in the late 1950s. The continuous monitoring of the electrocardiogram allows the staff to recognize when a patient develops arrhythmias that need either immediate treatment with antiarrhythmic drugs or cardioversion or should be studied in an electrophysiology laboratory.

Patients recovering from myocardial infarction who have ventricular premature beats or ventricular tachycardia and a badly damaged left ventricle are more likely to die sooner than those without such arrhythmias and relatively healthy left ventricles. Insertion of an implantable cardioverter defibrillator prophylactically can extend survival of such patients.

Three months later, the patient developed ventricular tachycardia that did not respond to pacing and the patient's defibrillator discharged for the first time. The episode occurred when he was at a movie. If the arrhythmia had progressed to ventricular fibrillation, he almost certainly would have died without the device to restore normal rhythm. He was told not to drive his car for up to 8 months after the episode, when the hazard of another dangerous cardiac event is highest. If he sustains ventricular tachycardia or fibrillation and loses consciousness while driving, he could have an accident before the defibrillator had restored normal cardiac function.

Now the doctor had to decide, given the two episodes, whether an antiarrhythmic drug should be given to reduce the likelihood of further episodes of ventricular tachycardia or fibrillation. Although the defibrillator would restore normal rhythm, each episode carried the risk of physical damage should he fall while standing or walking. As discussed with the previous patient, cardioverter-defibrillator usually treats ventricular tachycardia with pacing that the patient does not feel. If this fails, as was the case with this patient's ventricular tachycardia, or if the arrhythmia is ventricular fibrillation, then a shock will be delivered. Although life saving, shocks from an implantable cardioverter defibrillator hurt if the patient is conscious when the unit discharges and often alarm those near the patient. Furthermore, although infrequent, some damage to the heart can occur during the arrhythmia before the shock is delivered.

The doctor recommended that the patient take amiodarone, the antiarrhythmic drug that most cardiologists favor to reduce the frequency of dangerous ventricular arrhythmias in patients like this one. During the next year, the patient did not faint, and the defibrillator did not discharge.

This patient received his life-saving implantable cardioverter-defibrillator as prophylactic treatment for ventricular tachycardia or another episode of ventricular fibrillation. Unfortunately, most patients without implantable cardioverter defibrillators who sustain ventricular fibrillation will not be saved because help usually arrives after irreversible damage has occurred in the brain, heart, and other organs. If the potentially fatal arrhythmia had only happened during an acute myocardial infarction and if the patient had not developed ventricular tachycardia or ventricular premature beats afterwards, the chances of his having dangerous ventricular arrhythmias is much reduced, and a defibrillator might not have been prescribed.

Chapter 11

Heart Block in a 72-Year-Old Professor

While walking on a street near his home, this 72-year-old physics professor suddenly and unexpectedly became dizzy and fell to the ground. A neighbor ran to him and took his pulse, which seemed very slow. Gradually, the man awoke after being unconscious for about 30 seconds. His pulse rate increased, but never faster than 40 beats per minute. An ambulance was called, and he was brought to the emergency department of his local hospital.

By the time I saw him there, he was fully conscious and complaining of a sore left shoulder on which he had fallen. He told me that for several weeks before he fainted, he had felt weaker than usual and became short of breath walking up an incline and when climbing stairs. He was having difficulty concentrating when reading his professional literature and believed that his thinking processes were blunted.

His blood pressure was 140/60, but the values seemed to vary slightly from beat to beat. His pulse was regular at 40 beats per minute. In his neck, I saw abnormally large intermittent wave forms. On listening to his heart, I observed that the intensity of one of the heart sounds varied, as did that of a heart murmur, which when previously heard, had constant volume. The electrocardiogram showed complete heart block.

What Is Heart Block?

In heart block, the electrical signals originating in the sinus node, the heart's inherent pacemaker in the right atrium, do not reach the ventricles where the blood is pumped to the body. To keep the heart beating, subsidiary pacemakers in the ventricles take over and stimulate the heart. This backup system, however, does not do as good a job as the normal sinus node. The rate of these pacemakers in the ventricles is relatively slow, which means that less blood is ejected to the body each minute, accounting for the symptoms of weakness and shortness of breath during exertion. The brain may also receive less blood, and this can produce the neurological symptoms about which the patient complained.

In addition to discharging slower than the sinus node, the patient's ventricular pacemakers are less reliable and may stop functioning. When this happens, the heart stops beating, and no blood is sent to the brain and other parts of the body. After a few seconds, consciousness wanes, and the patient faints. In our patient, the reserve pacemakers started discharging again, and he recovered. If the ventricle does not start beating soon, however, the patient will die unless he receives immediate medical attention. Sometimes these episodes are caused by rapid, abnormal ventricular rhythms that can produce the same effect.

In complete heart block, the atria and ventricles beat independently, rather than in the normal sequence in which the atria contract first followed quickly by the ventricles. This asynchrony produces the physical signs I observed on examining the patient, the large pulsations in the neck, the varying intensity of the heart sounds and murmur, and the changes in the blood pressure. The large difference between the systolic pressure (the first number in the blood pressure reading) and the diastolic pressure (the second number) of 140/60 is caused by the very slow rate. Before he developed heart block, his blood pressure was 130/75.

Heart block is defined in three degrees. Our patient had third-degree block in which none of the atrial signals reached the ventricles, and the heart depends on subsidiary pacemakers to function. In second-degree block, some of the atrial stimuli reach the ventricles, and some do not. This produces an irregular heart rhythm, but the rate is usually faster than in third-degree block. In first-degree block, the atrial signals take longer to reach the ventricles than is normal, but none are blocked. First-degree block produces no symptoms, and the diagnosis is made on the electrocardiogram. Sometimes first-degree block progresses to higher degrees of block.

Symptoms

The most dramatic symptom associated with heart block is *syncope* (fainting).* The British cardiologist Paul Wood described such episodes with his characteristic flair:[9]

> Loss of consciousness is abrupt, without warning. If standing, the patient collapses, and lies limp, still, pale and pulseless, with fixed, dilated pupils—as if dead; breathing, however, continues. . . . As a rule . . . ventricular beating is resumed after a few seconds, consciousness returns abruptly, and a vivid flush ensues. When an attack occurs in bed, the lack of warning, short duration of unconsciousness, and abrupt return of full possession of the faculties, may prevent a dull patient from being aware of the fit, and he may only notice the flush. The sequence of events, both symptomatically and objectively, is so characteristic as to make the diagnosis probable on the history alone.

---

* These episodes are known as Adams-Stokes or Morgagni-Adams-Stokes attacks. Giovanni Batista Morgagni (1682–1771) was a Paduan physician who reported for the first time, in Latin, the scientific language of the day, the course of his friend, Father Poggi. Morgagni observed an episode when the priest fainted and had the wit to take his pulse, which was very slow. He treated him with bleeding and laudanum (opium) to no avail, and his friend eventually died. Robert Adams (1791–1875) was a Dublin surgeon who first described the syndrome in English, and William Stokes (1804–1878), an Irish physician, wrote about the unique physical findings that patients in heart block demonstrate.

Patients with heart block can have palpitations or become light-headed or dizzy. However, these symptoms occur so frequently and from so many different causes that they seldom provide doctors with the diagnosis. This requires that the patient be examined and an electrocardiogram taken.

As our patient experienced, the slow heart rate of complete heart block can decrease the function of the heart sufficiently to produce shortness of breath on exertion, weakness, faintness, and reduced brain function. Some patients with heart block develop congestive heart failure, in which the heart, unable to pump blood forward to the body adequately, allows the blood and its constituents to collect in the lungs and other parts of the body, adding to the shortness of breath and producing edema (collections of fluid) in different parts of the body. Patients with complete heart block, however, seldom have the chest pain of angina pectoris.

Causes of Heart Block

Healthy People

Even healthy people can have transient heart block without ill effect. First- and second-degree blocks frequently appear in well-trained athletes, particularly when they are resting. The block disappears soon after they stop training. Coughing, hiccups, swallowing, the Valsalva maneuver—even the sight of food in highly susceptible patients—occasionally produce transitory block, which can also appear in otherwise normal subjects when lying down. Normal rhythm returns when they stand or exercise. A few healthy adults develop first-, second-, and rarely third-degree atrioventricular block during sleep.

Fibrosis of Conducting Tissue

The most common cause of permanent heart block in older patients, like ours, is fibrosis of the conducting system. A process of unknown nature destroys the tissues that conduct electrical activity into and within the ventricles and replaces these tissues with fibrous material that cannot conduct electricity. We do not know much about this process or what causes it. Many patients with this disease have nothing else wrong with their hearts—no history of myocardial infarctions and no disease of the heart valves or significant hypertension. This is why, if they receive a pacemaker, their prognosis is no worse than in patients without heart block.

Myocardial Infarction

Complete heart block complicates the course of myocardial infarction in about 7% of cases. In general, these patients have had more heart damage and more complications such as other arrhythmias and congestive failure than patients without heart block. For reasons not well understood, heart block develops during myocardial infarction more frequently in women than men. Although temporary pacing may be needed if the heart rate falls to low rates, the heart block usually resolves as the patient recovers.

Cardiomyopathy

This cardiac disease, sometimes of unknown cause—it can be produced by alcohol in susceptible patients—converts functioning heart muscle into fibrous tissue that cannot contract. The eventual result is congestive heart failure. The process can also interfere with the conduction system and produce heart block.

Congenital Complete Heart Block

Occasionally, a child may develop heart block in utero and, when born, have a heart rate that is slower than is normal for an infant. An electrocardiogram will confirm that congenital complete heart block is present. The hearts of a majority of these children are otherwise normal, but some may have additional congenital abnormalities.

The mothers of about half of children with congenital complete heart block have connective tissue disease such as lupus erythematous. Most children born to women with lupus do not have heart block, however.

Valve Disease

Complete heart block occasionally develops in patients with such lesions as aortic stenosis, but this complication is rare. When the valves are infected with bacteria in the serious condition known as infective endocarditis, heart block can develop.

Lyme Disease

Probably the most common infective cause of heart block in the United States is Lyme disease caused by the organism *Borrelia burgdorferi*, which humans acquire from the bite of a tick. Patients with Lyme disease have, among other symptoms, fever, fatigue, malaise, and headache and a characteristic skin lesion called *erythema migrans*, which develops where the tick has bitten through the skin and introduced the organism. It is typically a painless, reddish lesion that gradually expands as the central portion clears and when present, as it usually is, strongly suggests the diagnosis.

When the infection affects the heart, which occurs in about 10% of patients with Lyme disease, the infection can produce heart block, which is complete in about half. With appropriate treatment of Lyme disease, the block almost always disappears.

Rheumatic Fever

This scourge, formerly a common cause of heart disease in the United States, often produces heart block during its acute phase.

Cardiac Surgery

Heart block sometimes complicates the postoperative course of patients who have had cardiac surgery. The block, however, is usually temporary and disappears without the need for a pacemaker.

Obstructive Sleep Apnea

Heart block sometimes develops in patients with this condition.

Treatment

I explained to the patient the nature of his problem and advised that he have an electronic pacemaker inserted. This device would return his heart rate to normal and relieve his symptoms. He accepted this approach, and the team performed the operation that afternoon.

The patient was taken to the electrophysiology laboratory. Electrocardiographic leads were attached to the patient to monitor his cardiac action, and he was given a mild sedative to relieve some of his anxiety. After preparing the skin of the chest and administering a local anesthetic, the doctors made a small incision in the left upper chest wall and created a pocket beneath the skin and muscles. They then located a large vein, opened it, and threaded the pacemaker's electrodes into the patient's heart while watching the scene on imaging equipment. One electrode was placed in the right ventricle and the other in the right atrium. The ends of the electrodes protruding from the wound were then connected to the pacemaker, which is only 2 inches wide (Figure 14-1). Before closing the skin and muscles over the pacemaker, the team checked the pacemaker to be sure that it would function as designed and then applied a bandage. The procedure took about 1 hour.

The patient went home the next morning. When he came to the office 2 weeks later, he reported that he felt normal and that the symptoms he had described while in heart block were gone. He had not fainted again.

The pacemaker that our patient and most patients with heart block receive replaces the slow, ventricular-driven heart rhythm with a faster rate. The electrode in the right atrium senses when the atrium discharges, inserts a brief pause, as normally occurs, and then stimulates the ventricles. As the sinus node increases or decreases its rate according to the patient's activities, the ventricles follow as they did before heart block developed.

Prognosis

Many patients with complete heart block have no other heart disease than the electrical disturbance. With a pacemaker, the prognosis for such a patient is the same as for someone without heart block. Before implantable pacemakers were developed in the late 1950s, half of patients with complete heart block died during the first year after the diagnosis was made.

The future may be less certain in patients with heart block whose ventricles have been affected by previous myocardial infarctions or by cardiomyopathy. With a pacemaker installed to treat the block, the prognosis will depend more on the severity of the associated heart disease than on the block.

Chapter 12

Sick Sinus Syndrome and Carotid Sinus Hypersensitivity in a 60-Year-Old Man

I was asked to consult on a 60-year-old lawyer who had been admitted to the hospital for resection of an abdominal aneurysm. The patient told me that on two or three occasions during the past month, most recently while walking in his garden, he became light-headed and dropped to the ground. He did not completely lose consciousness, was aware of what was happening, and was able to stand within seconds after falling. Because no one saw these episodes, we do not know what was the rate or rhythm of his pulse. The patient had no palpitations or awareness of any cardiac abnormality during the episodes.

Causes of Syncope

The suddenness of the onset and the recovery of the symptoms in this case are characteristic of a temporary change in the rhythm of his heart. They are not typical of *vasovagal syncope*, the most common cause of fainting. In this condition, which can occur in otherwise healthy people and seldom when they are recumbent, neurological stimuli dilate the blood vessels and often slow the heart rate thereby temporarily reducing the amount of blood in the ventricles and the flow of blood to the brain. Precipitating factors include pain—during such minor medical procedures as drawing blood, for example—trauma, fatigue, blood loss, or prolonged motionless standing as in soldiers at attention. Patients with vasovagal syncope may feel lightheaded, dizzy, sweaty, and nauseated, sense dimming of their vision and salivate before fainting. Observers often observe that patients about to faint with vasovagal syncope have become pale.

Another cause of syncope that doctors must consider is disease within the brain or the blood vessels supplying the brain. *Epilepsy* can produce unconsciousness, but this condition is almost always associated with neurological findings such as seizures, tongue biting, or involuntary passage of urine or stool. Normal mental function returns gradually after seizures, not almost at once as our patient experienced. A *stroke* occasionally causes patients to faint, but symptoms and findings of neurological damage will appear. Syncope rarely complicates *transient ischemic attacks* in which a portion of the brain is temporarily deprived of blood because of disease in an artery supplying the brain.

My examination of the patient's heart was normal, as was his electrocardiogram. I then applied pressure on his right carotid sinus.

The two carotid sinuses, located within the carotid arteries just below the jaw, regulate the blood pressure and the heart rate depending on the amount and pressure of the blood passing by them. They are richly supplied with autonomic nerves, the type not under voluntary control. External pressure on the carotid sinuses will slow the heart rate, in some cases abnormally in the condition known as carotid sinus hypersensitivity.

Before performing the test, I listened to his carotid arteries with my stethoscope to hear if a *bruit*, a murmur within the artery, was present, suggesting the presence of an obstruction within the vessel. Pressing on such vessels can release material into the circulation of the brain. No bruits were heard, and so I pressed gently on the right carotid sinus while simultaneously listened to his heart, and leaving the electrocardiogram running. Almost immediately the heart slowed and then stopped. I released the pressure. After 3 seconds, during which I must admit feeling some anxiety, the heart's beating gradually returned and rose to its normal rate. The patient told me that while I was pressing, he was beginning to have the symptoms that preceded one of his fainting episodes. I allowed the electrocardiogram to continue to run, and over the next 2 minutes, all cardiac electrical activity stopped for two periods of up to 2.5 seconds.

As his symptoms suggest, the cause of the patient's fainting is cardiovascular. He has carotid sinus hypersensitivity and the sick sinus syndrome. I demonstrated the first with carotid sinus pressure, and an episode of the second, captured on the electrocardiogram, appeared spontaneously soon afterward. The absence of any electrical activity, including the activation of the atria, established that the sinus node was periodically failing to discharge, producing the symptoms the patient described.

Both sick sinus syndrome and carotid sinus hypersensitivity are associated with advancing age. Few examples of either occur in patients less than 50 years of age. Men and women are equally affected. A majority of patients with sick sinus syndrome have such cardiac pathology as coronary heart disease or, less often, cardiomyopathy.

The physician, evaluating a patient with sick sinus syndrome, must review the drugs that he or she is taking, for several of them, often used for cardiac disease, can cause or more commonly exacerbate the manifestations of sick sinus syndrome. A frequent culprit is a beta blocker. It may slow the heart rate excessively in patients with sick sinus syndrome.

Some patients with sick sinus syndrome have abnormally rapid as well as slow heart rhythms, a variant known as the *tachycardia-bradycardia syndrome*. Examples of the tachyarrhythmias include atrial fibrillation, atrial flutter, and supraventricular tachycardia. Often the fainting occurs when the tachycardia stops. In such patients, the tachycardia has suppressed the sinus node, which recovers slowly producing periods when the heart does not beat.

Treatment

I explained to the patient that the examination had revealed the cause of his symptoms and advised him to have a pacemaker. He agreed. The instrument was installed that afternoon, and the patient was discharged the next day to recover from the procedure. He was readmitted a month later for the operation that had brought him to the hospital originally. He also recovered from this procedure without complications. When he came to my office 3 months later, he reported having no episodes of fainting. He has remained well during the ensuing 3 years.

We treat sick sinus syndrome and carotid sinus hypersensitivity with pacemakers, as you might expect. These devices will prevent the heart rate from falling below a rate that will assure normal cardiovascular function.

Sick sinus syndrome is one of the principal indications for the use of pacemakers. Not infrequently, however, the device does not cure the patient. I have seen several such cases, and each time, the diagnosis had been assumed but not established. The resting heart rate of the patient may be, for example, 45 or 50 per minute, and the doctor may assume that this indicates sick sinus syndrome. It may not.

As you can gather from this chapter, there are several causes of lightheadedness, dizziness, and fainting, many of which sound superficially like the sick sinus syndrome. Thus, before prescribing a pacemaker, the doctor should obtain proof that the symptoms are really due to the syndrome. Usually, the patient will not demonstrate this in the office or hospital, as this patient did. The physician must then use a device that will record the patient's electrocardiogram during his or her daily activities and try to document that the symptoms coincide with the appropriate electrocardiographic findings.

There is one very important limitation to this approach. In a patient with symptoms typical of sick sinus syndrome who has significant heart disease such as previous myocardial infarction or cardiomyopathy, the cause may be ventricular tachycardia or even ventricular fibrillation. Such patients must have an electrophysiological study because some may need an implantable cardioverter defibrillator rather than just a pacemaker.

Part III

Treating Arrhythmias

Chapter 13

Drugs Used to Treat Arrhythmias

Adenosine

Action

Adenosine (Adenocard) slows conduction in the A-V node (Table 13-1). It is given only intravenously and is metabolized very rapidly—half of the injection is inactivated in 10 seconds.

Indications

- *Supraventricular tachycardia.* Adenosine converts most patients with paroxysms of SVT to sinus rhythm. Because of its effectiveness and short duration of action, many doctors choose adenosine to convert SVT. If adverse reactions occur, they disappear quickly.
- *Atrial fibrillation and atrial flutter.* Adenosine does not convert these arrhythmias but, by slowing conduction in the A-V node, briefly decreases the ventricular rate. With the electrocardiogram showing a slower ventricular rate, the arrhythmia can be diagnosed more easily and appropriate definitive treatment instituted.

TABLE 13-1 Drugs Used to Treat Cardiac Arrhythmias

Generic name	Trade name	Indications	Cardiac side effects	Other side effects
Adenosine	Adenocard®	Supraventricular tachycardia Atrial fibrillation Atrial flutter	Slow heart rate Heart block Sick sinus syndrome	Facial flushing Shortness of breath Chest pressure
Amiodarone	Cardarone® Pacerone®	Premature beats (seldom) Atrial fibrillation Atrial flutter Supraventricular tachycardia Ventricular tachycardia Ventricular fibrillation	Proarrhythmia (can occasionally produce arrhythmias for which drug was prescribed)	Lung disease Photophobia Skin discoloration Thyroid dysfunction
Beta blockers Atenolol Esmolol Bisoprolol Metoprolol	*Beta blockers* Tenormin® Brevibloc® Zebeta® Lopressor® and Toprol-XL®	Premature beats Atrial fibrillation Atrial flutter Supraventricular tachycardia	Lower blood pressure Slow heart rate Decrease cardiac contractions Heart block Sick sinus syndrome	Tiredness Lightheadedness Depression Insomnia Worsen asthma

TABLE 13-1 Drugs Used to Treat Cardiac Arrhythmias (*continued*)

Generic name	Trade name	Indications	Cardiac side effects	Other side effects
Calcium blockers Diltiazem Verapamil	*Calcium blockers* Cardizem® Calan® Covera-HS® Isoptin® Verelan®	Supraventricular tachycardia Atrial fibrillation Atrial flutter	Lower blood pressure Slow heart rate Decrease cardiac contractions Heart block Sick sinus syndrome	Swelling of feet and legs Sinus congestion Rash Dreams Depression Loss of appetite Constipation Diarrhea
Propafenone	Rhythmol®	Atrial fibrillation Atrial flutter Ventricular tachycardia	Proarrhythmia Heart block Sick sinus syndrome	Unusual taste Nausea, vomiting Constipation Dizziness Headache Fatigue Weakness
Ibutilide	Carvert®	Atrial fibrillation Atrial flutter	Proarrhythmia Raise or lower blood pressure Heart block	Nausea Headache
Sotalol	Betapace®	Ventricular tachycardia Ventricular fibrillation	Proarrhythmia See Beta-blockers	See Beta-blockers

Cardiac Side Effects

These include transient slow heart rates, heart block, and sick sinus syndrome.

Other Side Effects

Facial flushing, shortness of breath, and chest pressure are among the most common. Occasionally headache, sweating, hyperventilation, light-headedness, dizziness, tingling, nausea, and metallic taste may occur.

Amiodarone

Amiodarone (Cordarone, Pacerone) is a particularly effective antiarrhythmic drug that has become a favorite choice of cardiologists in the treatment of many arrhythmias. Amiodarone is usually administered orally but can be given intravenously.

Amiodarone has some unusual properties and more than its share of side effects, particularly when large doses are prescribed. A few of these can be serious. Consequently, many doctors prefer to prescribe drugs they perceive to have fewer side effects, even though they may be less effective as antiarrhythmic drugs than amiodarone.

Indications

- *Premature beats.* Although seldom necessary to prescribe for this purpose, amiodarone is particularly effective in suppressing premature beats.
- *Atrial fibrillation and flutter.* Despite its side effects, amiodarone is probably the most effective drug to prevent episodes of these arrhythmias. Given orally or intravenously during paroxysms of the arrhythmias, amiodarone will slow the ventricular rate and, in some cases, convert the heart to normal rhythm.
- *SVT.* Because of its nearly universal slowing effect on conduction, amiodarone given intravenously converts most episodes of SVT whether sustained within the atrioventricular node or an accessory

pathway. The drug also reduces the number of paroxysms of the arrhythmia. Other drugs, such as adenosine, however, are similarly effective and are usually chosen for conversion and suppression because they produce fewer side effects. Ablation is the preferred treatment for chronic suppression.

- *Ventricular tachycardia and ventricular fibrillation.* Amiodarone, despite its side effects, is the best drug to treat these dangerous arrhythmias in most patients. Even in those whose ventricles are badly diseased from myocardial infarction or cardiomyopathy, amiodarone is less likely than most other antiarrhythmic drugs to induce additional, potentially fatal arrhythmias. Most patients with ventricular tachycardia and all patients resuscitated from ventricular fibrillation will also receive implantable cardioverter defibrillators.

Slow Onset

Unlike most drugs used for treating heart disease, amiodarone takes a long time to work and, conversely, to leave the body when it is stopped. Accordingly, doctors must load the patient with large amounts of the drug for as long as is necessary to achieve suppression of the arrhythmia. Typically, patients take 400 milligrams (two 200-milligram tablets) three times a day for a week or more. When effective levels are reached, the dose is usually decreased to 100 or 200 milligrams once per day.

Slow Removal

The liver and kidney do not metabolize (break down into inactive substances) or excrete amiodarone as they do for most drugs. Amiodarone leaves the body in rejected cells of the skin and gastrointestinal tract but takes weeks or even months to be eliminated. If one must stop taking amiodarone, its effects can continue for a long time.

Cardiac Side Effects

The most serious side effect that amiodarone can produce is *proarrhythmia* in which the drug produces ventricular tachycardia, *torsades de pointes* (a variant of ventricular tachycardia) or ventricular fibrillation despite its having been given to suppress these arrhythmias. The more damaged the ventricles are by such diseases as myocardial infarction or cardiomyopathy, the more likely proarrhythmia will occur. Of all of the antiarrhythmic drugs available to suppress ventricular tachycardia and ventricular fibrillation, however, amiodarone is the least likely to produce serious arrhythmias.

Amiodarone can exacerbate atrioventricular block and sick sinus syndrome in patients with a tendency for these problems.

Other Side Effects

- *Lung.* The most serious non-cardiac problem with amiodarone is its occasional production of lung disease, which, if not detected in time, can be fatal. The disease, called *hypersensitivity* or *interstitial/ alveolar pneumonitis,* is more likely to occur in patients regularly taking large doses of the drug, such as 400 or more milligrams per day. The course of the complication may be more severe in those who already have lung disease. The disease produces coughing, difficulty breathing, fever, and malaise, which may develop insidiously or suddenly. If these symptoms appear, the patient should tell the doctor immediately. After the diagnosis is confirmed—much less serious conditions, of course, can produce coughing, malaise, and fever—the amiodarone is stopped, and if the findings are marked, patients may be given corticosteroid drugs to encourage healing. Doctors often hospitalize patients with this condition until resolution begins.
- *Skin.* Many patients find that they respond more quickly to the effects of sunlight with early tanning and burning (*photosensitivity*) when taking amiodarone. Patients should stay out of bright sunlight whenever possible and use sunscreen when appropriate. Another unique effect of the drug is discoloration of the skin with a bluish gray tint, particularly when the drug is taken in high doses and for prolonged periods of time. Sunlight can worsen this effect. This problem, of cosmetic importance only, may slowly disappear when the drug is stopped.
- *Thyroid.* Because amiodarone contains large amounts of iodine—an element that the thyroid gland stores—the drug can occasionally pro-

duce *hypothyroidism* or *hyperthyroidism* (thyrotoxicosis). Each of these complications can be successfully treated, and in some cases, the patient may continue to take amiodarone. Doctors caring for patients on amiodarone order blood tests of thyroid function periodically to check for these problems.

- *Liver.* The liver function tests of some patients taking relatively large doses of amiodarone may become abnormal. Clinical liver disease rarely results, and consequently, the drug may often be continued as the liver tests are followed.
- *Eye.* Tiny deposits in the cornea of the eye can be detected in most patients taking amiodarone for more than about 6 months. Unless vision is affected, which is rare, the drug need not be discontinued.

Beta-Adrenergic Blocking Drugs

These drugs, most commonly used for treating hypertension, can also treat arrhythmias effectively.

Action

Beta-adrenergic blocking drugs compete with the effects of the beta-adrenergic nervous system, which in the heart speeds the rate and increases the force of contraction. Beta-1-selective, also called cardioselective, agents have fewer effects on organs other than the heart. Examples include atenolol (Tenormin), esmolol (Brevibloc), bisoprolol (Zebeta), and metoprolol (Lopressor and Toprol-XL).

Indications

- *Premature beats.* Beta-blocking drugs are often prescribed first when premature beats need specific treatment. They suppress the beats in some patients or make the beats less noticeable by decreasing the strength of ventricular contraction.
- *Atrial fibrillation and atrial flutter.* These drugs decrease the heart (ventricular) rate by slowing conduction within the A-V node.

- *SVT.* Beta blockers convert many episodes of SVT by slowing conduction in one of the pathways sustaining the arrhythmia. They may also reduce the frequency of episodes of or eliminate the arrhythmia completely.

Cardiac Side Effects

Because beta-blocking drugs decrease the force of ventricular contraction, they can lower the blood pressure. Accordingly, hypertension is one of the leading indications for these drugs. In diseased hearts, however, the drugs can so decrease the cardiac function that congestive heart failure or hypotension may develop. These serious effects seldom occur. Because beta-blocking drugs slow conduction in the A-V node, they may worsen atrioventricular block due to pathology in the node. They also decrease the discharge rate of the sinus node and, consequently, may exacerbate sick sinus syndrome in patients with slow sinus rhythms.

Other Side Effects

Tiredness and lightheadedness are among the most frequent. Some patients note mental depression with insomnia and vivid dreams. Asthma may appear or worsen, particularly in patients with this disease. Beta-adrenergic blocking drugs cause fewer problems in noncardiac organs when one of the cardioselective versions is prescribed.

Calcium-Channel Blocking Drugs

Action

Those calcium-channel blocking drugs that affect cardiac electrophysiological function interfere with the action of calcium ions,* which are essential for normal conduction in the A-V node.

---

* Calcium ions are important participants in many biological functions. In its pure form, calcium is a metallic, silvery white element. It does not occur naturally this way but is usually combined with other elements. An ion is a form of an element that has lost or acquired an electron.

Indications

- *SVT.* The calcium-channel blocking drug most frequently given intravenously to convert SVT is diltiazem (Cardizem). Verapamil is also effective. The same drugs, given orally, can reduce the likelihood of recurrent attacks.
- *Atrial fibrillation and atrial flutter.* These drugs decrease the ventricular rate by blocking transmission of atrial signals through the atrioventricular node.

Cardiac Side Effects

Like beta-adrenergic blocking drugs, calcium-channel blocking drugs will slow the normal heart rate, can produce heart block and worsen sick sinus syndrome. Calcium-channel blocking drugs are commonly used to treat hypertension and may decrease the blood pressure too much in certain patients. The drugs must be given with care to patients with decreased heart function because they can produce or worsen congestive heart failure.

When drugs are given intravenously for conversion of an arrhythmia such as SVT, a defibrillator should always be available in case another arrhythmia develops or the blood pressure drops. These problems seldom occur.

Other Side Effects

Edema (swelling) of the feet and legs, sinus congestion, rash, abnormal dreams, depression, loss of appetite, constipation, and diarrhea can occur.

Propafenone (Rhythmol)

Action

This antiarrhythmic drug is prescribed to suppress paroxysmal (episodic) arrhythmias.

Indications

- *Atrial fibrillation and atrial flutter.* Propafenone suppresses paroxysms of these arrhythmias in many patients.

- *SVT.* Propafenone suppresses recurrence of SVT in some patients.
- *Ventricular tachycardia.* Propafenone suppresses recurrences of sustained ventricular tachycardia in some patients. Because of its tendency for proarrhythmia, patients being given propafenone should be observed in a monitoring unit when the drug is started. Amiodarone and sotalol are more frequently used for this arrhythmia.

Cardiac Side Effects

It can worsen sick sinus syndrome, heart block, and congestive failure and may increase the ventricular rate in some patients with atrial flutter. It can produce dangerous arrhythmias (proarrhythmia), particularly in patients with reduced ventricular function.

Other Side Effects

Unusual taste, nausea or vomiting, constipation, dizziness, headache, fatigue, and weakness can occur. Propafenone can worsen chronic bronchitis and emphysema and has been rarely reported to produce agranulocytosis in which the cells producing red blood cells, white cells, and platelets malfunction. This complication usually resolves when the drug is stopped. Propafenone should be given with particular care to patients with liver or kidney disease.

Ibutilide (Corvert)

Action

This is an antiarrhythmic drug with properties that are similar to amiodarone and sotalol. Ibutilide is only given by intravenous infusion.

Indications

- *Atrial Fibrillation and Atrial Flutter.* Ibutilide converts many paroxysms of these arrhythmias if they started recently. The drug is less effective in converting chronic, long established arrhythmias.

If ibutilide does not convert the arrhythmia, the next treatment is usually cardioversion. The drug, given, with cardioversion, may improve the likelihood that normal rhythm will be established.

Cardiac Side Effects

Ibutilide can produce new arrhythmias (proarrhythmia), increase or decrease the blood pressure, and may worsen heart block. Consequently, ibutilide is not usually given to patients with significant heart disease other than the arrhythmia for which it is prescribed.

Other Side Effects

These include nausea and headache.

Sotalol (Betapace)

Action

Sotalol has antiarrhythmic properties similar to those of amiodarone plus some beta-adrenergic blocking actions. These effects, however, are not cardioselective, and the drug can influence beta-adrenergic responses in organs other than the heart. Because, like amiodarone, sotalol can have serious side effects, most physicians use the drug only for dangerous ventricular arrhythmias. Patients being started on sotalol should be observed in a cardiac monitoring unit for several days.

Indications

- *Ventricular tachycardia and ventricular fibrillation.* Sotalol, like amiodarone, suppresses dangerous ventricular arrhythmias in many patients. All patients being treated for ventricular tachycardia should also have an implantable cardioverter defibrillator for protection against developing ventricular fibrillation.
- *Other arrhythmias.* Because of its proarrhythmic effects, sotalol is seldom prescribed for patients with less serious tachyarrhythmias such

as atrial fibrillation, atrial flutter, or SVT, even if the patients are symptomatic. Similarly, sotalol is not prescribed for patients with ventricular premature beats whether or not the arrhythmia is producing symptoms.

Cardiac Side Effects

Sotalol, like all antiarrhythmic drugs, can produce the arrhythmias it has been given to suppress such as ventricular tachycardia or ventricular fibrillation. The more damaged the ventricles by such diseases as myocardial infarction or cardiomyopathy, the more likely sotalol will produce proarrhythmia.

Other Antiarrhythmic Drugs

Digitalis, procainamide (Pronestyl), and quinidine, the only drugs available for treatment of arrhythmias several decades ago, are seldom prescribed for this purpose now.

Chapter 14

Devices Used to Treat Arrhythmias

Pacemakers

Pacemakers are used to treat slow heart rhythms, called *bradyarrhythmias* in medical jargon. By stimulating the atria and ventricles, they establish a rhythm that simulates the normal condition. Heart block and sick sinus syndrome are the principal indications.

Current models (called pulse generators) are very compact—only 2 inches wide and 0.25-inch thick (Figure 14-1)—making them barely noticeable when implanted under the skin of the upper chest (Figure 14-2). The electrical impulses are generated in the pacemaker itself, and the signals are transmitted to the heart through electrode catheters attached in the plastic device at the top of the pacemaker. One electrode is passed through a vein in the chest into the right ventricle to stimulate the ventricles (Figure 14-2A). Often a second electrode is guided into the right atrium, where it senses atrial electrical activity, and when indicated, paces the atria as well (Figure 14-2B). The units only need to be replaced in about 10 years.

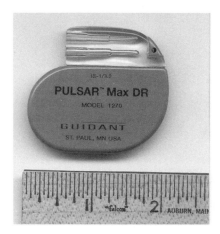

FIGURE 14-1   Cardiac Pacemaker

In heart block, the pacemaker can sense, through the atrial electrode, how fast the sinus node wants the heart to beat and then pace the ventricles at that rate through the ventricular electrode. In sick sinus syndrome, the atrial electrode will drive the heart when the sinus node cannot produce a heart rate adequate for the body's requirements.

Contemporary pacemakers have the ability to sense when a faster heart rate is needed, during exercise, for example, and then pace the heart at a faster rate than when the patient is resting.

Implantable Cardioverter Defibrillator

By shocking or pacing the ventricles, implantable cardioverter defibrillators restore normal rhythm in patients with ventricular tachycardia or ventricular fibrillation. Like pacemakers, implantable cardioverter defibrillators are inserted under the skin of the upper chest, and electrodes are passed through veins in the chest to the heart chambers. Current models of implantable cardioverter defibrillators are not much larger than pacemakers (Figure 14-3).

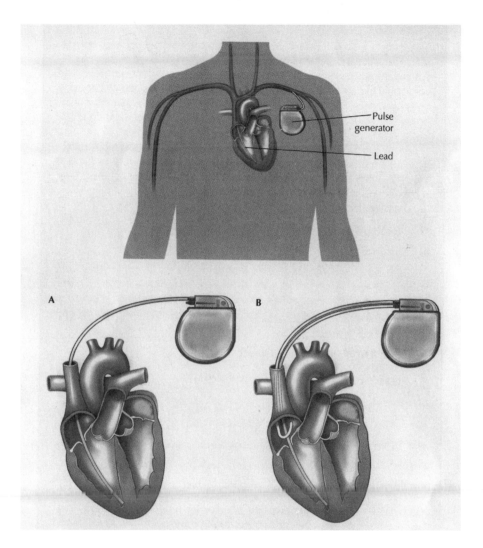

Pulse
generator

Lead

A

B

FIGURE 14-2   Pacemaker in the Body

Implantable cardioverter-defibrillators can terminate many episodes of ventricular tachycardia by pacing—all contemporary defibrillators can also function as pacemakers. When pacing is unsuccessful or in ventricular fibrillation, an arrhythmia that cannot be converted by pacing, the unit delivers shocks that re-establish normal rhythm.

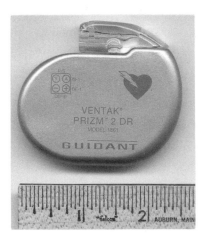

FIGURE 14-3   Implantable Cardioverter-Defibrillator

Part IV

The Electrocardiogram

Chapter 15

The Machine

The electrocardiogram is the tool that doctors use to evaluate the electrical activity of the heart and diagnose arrhythmias. It shows the electrical activation, not the mechanical action, of the atria and ventricles as they contract and recover. The electrocardiogram does not detect the signals that travel from sinus node to atrioventricular node to bundle of His through the bundle branches to the ventricles because the electrical potentials they generate are too weak for the clinical electrocardiogram machine to record.

The electrocardiogram machine uses 12 *leads* to record the heart's electrical information. The device electronically selects and then prints the leads sequentially from 10 wires attached to plastic electrodes that are placed at specific locations on the patient's limbs and chest. The leads give different views of the heart's electrical activity and guided doctors in analyzing many aspects of the heart's electrical function (Table 15-1).

The deflections on the electrocardiogram corresponding to the activation of the atria are called *P waves* and of the ventricles *QRS complexes*. The *T waves* reflect the electrophysiological recovery of the ventricles after they contract (Figure 15-1).*

---

* The familiar P-QRS-T nomenclature is almost 100 years old. It was devised by Wilhelm Einthoven, the Dutch physician–scientist who won the Nobel Prize in physiology or medicine in 1924 for developing the clinical electrocardiogram.[10]

TABLE 15-1   The Leads of the Electrocardiogram

Lead	Location
I	Left arm and right arm
II	Right arm and left leg
III	Left leg and left arm
aV_r	Right arm versus left arm and left leg
aV_l	Left arm versus right arm and left leg
aV_f	Left leg versus left arm and right arm
V_1	Fourth interspace just to right of sternum
V_2	Fourth interspace just to left of sternum
V_3	Midway between V2 and V4
V_4	Fifth left interspace in midclavicular line
V_5	Fifth left interspace in anterior axillary line
V_6	Fifth left interspace in midaxillary line

Interspace = the indentation between ribs

Sternum = the bone that lies in the center of the chest (breastbone)

Midclavicular line = a vertical line (imaginary) drawn from the middle of the clavicle (collarbone)

Anterior axillary line = a vertical line drawn from the front of the axilla (armpit)

Midaxillary line = a vertical line drawn from the middle of the axilla

Leads I, II and III are called *bipolar leads*, and leads aV_r, aV_l, and aV_f are called *augmented unipolar limb leads*. The V leads are unipolar leads and are designed to be electrically positive. The lead on the right leg is electrically neutral.

The electrocardiogram paper contains vertical and horizontal lines. The vertical lines record time. With the paper traveling at a speed of 25 millimeters per second, the interval between two of the closest, thinnest lines is 40 milliseconds or 0.04 (1/25) seconds. Each group of five of these lines is grouped together by thicker lines at 200 milliseconds or 0.2 (1/5) second intervals. To determine the rate, divide 60 by the time between two neighboring identical deflections, such as between two adjacent QRS complexes. For example, 60 ÷ 1.00 seconds = 60 beats per minute; 60 ÷ 0.60 seconds = 100 beats per minute; 60 ÷ 0.4 seconds = 150 beats per minute. Fortunately, for doctors reading electrocardio-

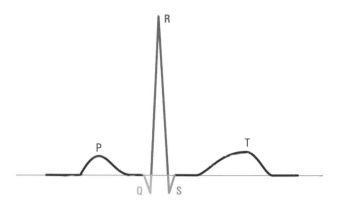

FIGURE 15-1   P, QRS, and T Waves

grams, computers automatically perform this arithmetic and print the rates on the tracing!

The horizontal lines record the strength of the electrical signals detected by the machine. The distance between two thick horizontal lines or 10 thin lines corresponds to one millivolt of potential detected on the surface of the body in the lead examined.

In studying arrhythmias, we concentrate on the information the electrocardiogram provides with respect to time (vertical lines) rather than voltage (horizontal lines.)

Ambulatory Electrocardiographic Recording

The electrocardiogram will not provide a diagnosis if no arrhythmia occurs while the tracing is being taken. To overcome this limitation, devices are available that record the electrocardiogram when the patient is not in the laboratory.

The most frequently used technique, the *Holter monitor*,* is a compact cassette tape recorder that continuously registers the electrocardiogram for 24 to 48 hours. The patient keeps a diary of symptoms, if any. The doctor then analyzes the tape for the presence of arrhythmias and compares

---

* Named for Dr. Norman Holter, its inventor.

these data with the patient's diary. Not infrequently, the patient records having palpitations when the tape shows normal rhythm. The sensation, in such cases, is not due to an arrhythmia. Conversely, the tape may reveal the presence of arrhythmias when the patient has no symptoms.

The *patient-activated event monitor* is a small device that the patient triggers when sensing the presence of an arrhythmia. This method enables the doctor to evaluate arrhythmias, which may recur less frequently than would be recorded on a Holter monitor. The electrocardiogram can then be transmitted over the telephone or, in some cases, by wireless to a center where the signals are recorded for analysis.

The *implantable loop recorder* is surgically installed under the skin. The doctor can program it to record automatically abnormal fast and slow rhythms, or the patient can activate it by passing a small transmitter over the device when an arrhythmia is sensed. These compact devices are designed for patients with infrequent or short-lived episodes.

Many pacemakers and implantable defibrillators automatically record arrhythmias that will be revealed during electronic interrogation of the unit. If a patient needs one of these devices, however, an arrhythmia will usually have been diagnosed previously.

Other Cardiology Tests

Occasionally, the physician may order a stress test to confirm the diagnosis of an arrhythmia, particularly if the patient reports that the symptoms coincide with exercise or stress. The stress test can also indicate whether coronary artery disease contributes to the arrhythmia.

The doctor may order an echocardiogram to evaluate the mechanical function of the heart of a patient with an arrhythmia. This test reveals how well the ventricles contract and whether the valves are operating normally. Nuclear studies can also evaluate ventricular function.

Chapter 16

Electrocardiograms of Arrhythmias

Here are examples of electrocardiograms from patients with the arrhythmias described earlier in this book. Readers may be surprised how easy it is to recognize which arrhythmia is illustrated. Electrocardiography is much less complicated than you may think.

Normal Sinus Rhythm

The heart's normal rhythm originates in the sinus node and is consequently called *normal sinus rhythm* (Figure 16-1). The normal rate in a resting subject is conventionally defined as 60 to 100 beats per minute.

Sinus Tachycardia

When the heart beats more than 100 per minute from acceleration of the sinus node, the rhythm is called *sinus tachycardia* (Figure 16-2).

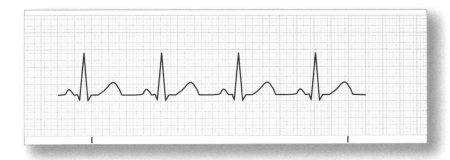

FIGURE 16-1   Normal Sinus Rhythm

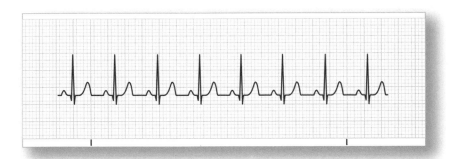

FIGURE 16-2   Sinus Tachycardia

Sinus Bradycardia

When the heart beats less than 60 beats per minute from slowing of the sinus node, the rhythm is called *sinus bradycardia* (Figure 16-3). Sinus bradycardia is frequently present when one is resting or taking drugs that slow the heart. The normal rate for resting well trained athletes is usually less than 60 beats per minute.

Ventricular Premature Beat

Ventricular premature beats originate in the ventricles, the principal pumping chambers of the heart. In Figure 16-4, we see two sinus beats

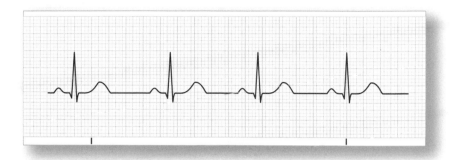

FIGURE 16-3   Sinus Bradycardia

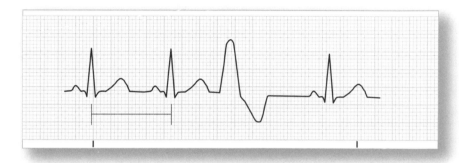

FIGURE 16-4   Ventricular Premature Beat

followed by a ventricular premature beat, which we recognize by its abnormally shaped, wide form and its appearance earlier than expected. Notice that the form in the premature beat of both the QRS complex (the positive deflection) and the T-wave (the negative deflection) are very different from in the four sinus beats. These characteristics reflect the beat's origin within the ventricles.

Atrial Fibrillation

We recognize atrial fibrillation by the irregularity of the ventricular rhythm and the replacement of formed P waves by *f waves*, undulations between the QRS complexes produced by the uncoordinated fibrillatory activity of the atria (Figure 16-5).

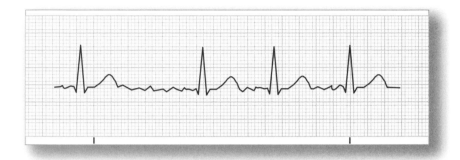

FIGURE 16-5   Atrial Fibrillation

Supraventricular Tachycardia (SVT)

The heart rate is rapid during SVT. In the example, the rate is about 166 beats per minute (60 ÷ 0.36) (Figure 16-6). The QRS complexes are characteristically normal, but P waves may not be seen. The deflections between the QRS complexes are T waves, not P waves.

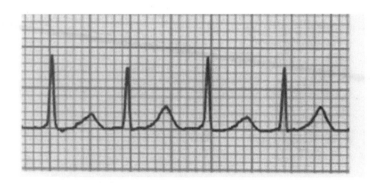

FIGURE 16-6   Supraventricular Tachycardia

Wolff-Parkinson-White Syndrome (W-P-W Syndrome)

The electrocardiogram of a patient with the Wolff-Parkinson-White syndrome when in normal rhythm shows short P-R intervals and delta waves. The P-R interval in Figure 16-7 is 0.08 seconds (two small horizontal boxes). The normal minimal P-R interval in adults is 0.12 seconds. The delta wave is the slurring in the upstroke of the QRS complex. As is often the case, the T-waves are abnormal; they should be upright in this lead.

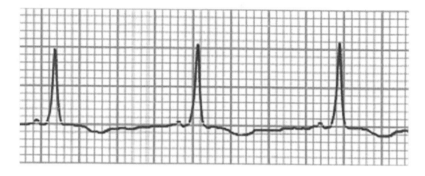

FIGURE 16-7   Wolff-Parkinson-White Syndrome (Type A)

Atrial Flutter

Flutter waves look like a picket fence or the teeth of a saw. The ventricular rhythm may be regular as in Figure 16-8 or irregular.

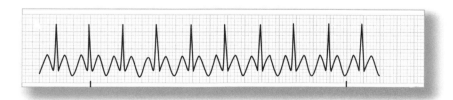

FIGURE 16-8   Atrial Flutter

Multifocal Atrial Tachycardia (MAT)

In multifocal atrial tachycardia, the P waves have several forms as they have in this example (Figure 16-9). The rhythm of the heart with multifocal atrial tachycardia is irregular.

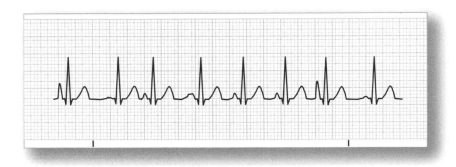

FIGURE 16-9   Multifocal Atrial Tachycardia

Ventricular Tachycardia

Because ventricular tachycardia originates in the ventricles, the QRS complexes look like a series of ventricular premature beats. The rate in Figure 16-10 from lead V$_1$ is about 170 beats per minute.

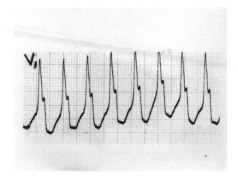

FIGURE 16-10   Ventricular Tachycardia

Ventricular Fibrillation

The electrocardiogram during ventricular fibrillation shows no QRS complexes, just disorganized electrical activity (Figure 16-11).

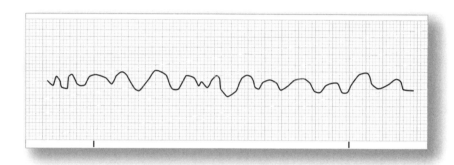

FIGURE 16-11   Ventricular Fibrillation

Complete Heart Block

Because no electrical signals pass between atria and ventricles in complete heart block, the QRS complexes (large deflections) and P waves (small deflections) bear no temporal relation to each other (Figure 16-12). P waves may be difficult to identify in a complete heart block. The ventricles are driven by subsidiary pacemakers in those chambers.

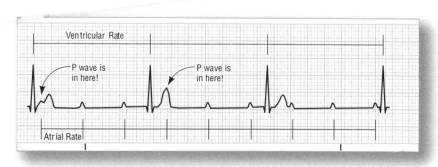

FIGURE 16-12   Complete Heart Block

Sick Sinus Syndrome

When the sinus node fails to discharge in patients with the sick sinus syndrome, the electrocardiogram shows no P waves or QRS complexes, and the heart does not beat. In Figure 16-13, the long period of *asystole* in which the heart is not beating lasts about 6 seconds.

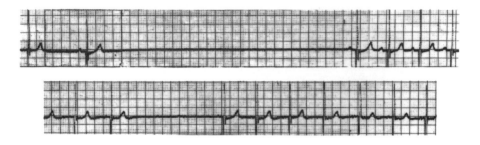

FIGURE 16-13   Sick Sinus Syndrome

Part V

Historical Reports

Chapter 17

Michel Mirowski and the Implantable Cardioverter-Defibrillator*

In one of the operating rooms at the Johns Hopkins Hospital in Baltimore, Maryland, a large group of people crowded the floor and the overhead viewing booth on February 4, 1980, to watch the first installation of an automatic implantable defibrillator in a human. The patient was a 57-year-old woman who had had a myocardial infarction and coronary artery bypass graft operation for angina. She had lost consciousness several times from ventricular tachycardia and fibrillation, and antiarrhythmic drugs had not controlled her symptoms. A fatal outcome from a future episode seemed inevitable. She had flown to Hopkins from California for the procedure with her cardiologist, Dr. Roger Winkle of Stanford University Medical School.

The operation was performed by Dr. Levi Watkins, a young Hopkins cardiothoracic surgeon. Assisting him was Dr. Philip R. Reed, a cardiac electrophysiologist and head of the arrhythmia service at Hopkins, and

---

* Adapted from Kastor JA. *Arrhythmias,* 2nd ed. Philadelphia: W.B. Saunders, 2000, chapter 2.[11]

Dr. Morton Mower, a cardiologist from Sinai Hospital of Baltimore and one of the developers of the defibrillator. Close to the operating table, in unaccustomed surgical scrub suit and mask, was Dr. Michel Mirowski, at 55 years of age the man whose waking hours had been dominated by his efforts to build the electronic device now being applied for the first time to treat a patient.

Michel Mirowski (Figure 17-1) believed that he began learning how to construct the automatic implantable defibrillator when he was 15 years old. At that time, there were no pacemakers, no external defibrillators, no clear understanding, in fact, of how to resuscitate a patient from cardiac arrest and Mirowski was certainly not considering then how to invent a defibrillator. However, he was about to have experiences that would teach him how to accomplish what seemed impossible.

Mieczyslaw (Michel) Mirowski was born Mordechai Friedman, the son of Israel Lieb Friedman and Genia Handelsman Friedman, on October 14, 1924, in Warsaw, Poland. His parents operated a delicatessen where much of the kosher food they sold was manufactured. "My parents worked long hours," he recalled. "I don't think my father ever took a vacation. My mother and I would leave Warsaw for a week or so in the summer and stay in a *pension* outside the city."

Warsaw was then a city of 1 million people, one third of whom, including the Mirowski family, were Jewish. Earlier generations of the family had been quite religious, but his parents' attitude was less orthodox, his father somewhat more traditional than his mother. Michel Mirowski, although deeply aware of his cultural heritage, was never religious.

Mirowski and many Warsaw Jews found the Polish culture attractive and tried to enter the more general Polish life. For this reason, Mirowski did not learn Yiddish as a boy even though the family spoke Yiddish as well as Polish in the home. His father had been raised speaking only

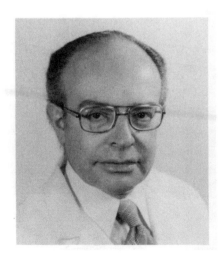

FIGURE 17-1   Michel Mirowski, MD

Yiddish, and Mirowski's paternal grandfather could probably speak no Polish at all. Later, to honor the traditions of his family, he learned to speak and write the language well.

Mirowski's mother's sister had become a lawyer, a significant accomplishment for a woman and a Jew in the Poland of the 1920s. The members of Mirowski's own and his father's generations would have had slightly less difficulty becoming members of the professional class because all were boys. When Mirowski and his wife later had daughters, a "family tradition" was broken.

To Mirowski and his family and to many of Poland's 3 to 4 million Jews—the total population of Poland in the early 1930s was about 30,000,000—their country seemed conservative, almost fascist, and definitely anti-Semitic. He remembered, "Even the police were sympathetic to right-wing trends. They stood aside when fascistic toughs beat and even killed Jews, and this was before the Nazis arrived."

The traditional restrictions still applied to the education of Jews. A *numerus clausus* limited the number who could study at the universities. Those Jews who were admitted had to sit in a special part of the classrooms. Rather than do so, many stood during the lectures.

Mirowski's formal education started at the age of 7 years when he began attending a Jewish private school because of the limited access to the public schools of Warsaw. The classes were taught in Polish. By 11 years old, he was in a private gymnasium, a school that prepared brighter students for the university. "We studied French, Latin and Hebrew. We read Sholom Aleichem in Polish, not in the Yiddish that Aleichem used," Mirowski remembered, "Though his work was obviously fine literature, I could not then relate myself to it, set, as the stories were, in the rural *shtetls*. In view of my career, it was probably significant that I was attracted to Paul de Kruif's *Microbe Hunters*. But the book which always seemed to have the greatest influence on me was *Martin Eden* by Jack London."[4]

In *Martin Eden*, written in 1909 when the author was 33 years old, London tells much about himself, a self-taught working man, deeply distressed by the effects of poverty and the life of the laborer. Eden, who supports himself, as London did, as a sailor and laborer, falls in love with Ruth, the college-educated daughter of an Oakland, California lawyer. She teaches him how to speak properly and what to learn to become a member of her class, to which he always feels an outsider.

Martin has a talent for writing, and after years of repeated rejections, his work is finally published, but when he becomes famous and acceptable to Ruth's parents, he rejects the life they offer, becomes increasingly depressed, goes back to sea, this time as a first-class passenger, slips out of his cabin porthole, and drowns himself.

It was Martin Eden, the outsider who succeeded, that appealed to Mirowski. He also saw himself able, by self-discipline and application of his own abilities, to overcome the most degrading difficulties. Eden's resolution to his conflicts, however, would never be suitable for Mirowski.

By September 1938, Mirowski was almost 14 years old and aware of the great political events occurring in Europe. The Munich settlement was followed 1 year later by the von Ribbentrop-Molotov nonaggression pact, which provided the political terms leading to the simultaneous German invasion of Poland from the West and Russian assault from the East.

His family survived the bombing of Warsaw, which opened World War II in September, 1939, but by 1945, only he would be alive.

> Six of the 30 members of my high school class, all boys of course, survived the war and the Holocaust, which is rather surprising. Some even got out with their families. We stay in contact. Two are in New York City, two in Paris, one in Geneva, and I am here in Baltimore. How did we make it? More luck than intelligence, probably, but good sense didn't hurt. Each of us has had a rather successful career, so stress and adversity need not necessarily have a negative effect.

In November, 1939, his mother, who was only 34 years old, died of heart failure. On December 1, all Jews were ordered to wear yellow stars on their clothes to identify themselves to the occupying Germans.

> When the war started, I had a liberal view of the world which was in conflict with the traditional Jewish reality in Poland. I thought I was, first of all, Polish—obviously a mistaken impression. I was committed, even then, to a life of study and education.
>
> Then the Nazis came. The schools were closed, and the persecution began. I remember German officers cutting off the *payess* [the long hair traditionally worn by Orthodox Jewish men] to humiliate them. I told my father that I wouldn't wear the yellow star and that it seemed foolish to stay in Warsaw. Worse things were obviously coming—although I can't say that I imagined what was really ahead. I had to continue my education since I knew I had some contribution to make although I had no idea

what it would be. Even then, I felt that I could overcome all difficulties. This was, and is, an irrational idea. In retrospect, it seems completely crazy that at the age of 15, I should leave my family, my town and my country.

At this point, his father gave him a new name in the hope that the change would help protect him from the deadly anti-Semitism of the time. Mordechai Friedman, now Mieczyslaw Mirowski—later, his wife, Anna, would call him Michel, by which name he would become known—would never see his father or younger brother Abraham again.

Escape and Survival

On December 5, Mirowski started east toward Russia. He traveled with a friend, heading toward Lvov, about 200 miles from Warsaw. Another friend of his had relatives there. They walked, rode in trucks and trains, and slept in railroad stations. Many days they spent the days in trenches, traveling at night to avoid capture. In Lvov, Mirowski lived in a house for war victims. Lvov had been incorporated into the Soviet Union soon after the beginning of World War II. Although Ukrainian was still the official language and much Polish was spoken there, Mirowski began learning Russian.

Lvov had been part of Poland since 1340 and by the end of the 14th century was the most important and populous Polish city. Later it would be ruled by the Swedes, the Austrians, the Russians, and briefly after World War I the Ukrainian nationalists. Lvov was one of the first large cities to fall to the Germans after their attack to the east in June 1941. The Russians recovered it in July 1944 and transferred most of the resident Poles to western Poland. The Jews, who built their first synagogue there in 1582, had been annihilated. Early in the 20th century, they had constituted almost one third of the population.

While Mirowski was in Lvov, the Soviet government ruled that refugees from German-conquered territories must live in cities and villages with populations of less than 100,000, which were at least 100 kilometers from the front. Refugees were expected to carry passports, but most did not want them because they feared that accepting passports would acknowledge possession of Russian citizenship. Those who were caught without passports were exiled to Siberia, many to labor camps.

Mirowski recalled this:

In July 1940, I was arrested by an officer whom I presumed at the time to be a general from the NKVD, the secret police. He seemed, to my eyes, so powerful that he *must* have been a general. I told him that I wasn't yet 16 years old and—such *chutzpah*—was too young to be issued a passport. It is true that I was 3 months short of my 16th birthday, but I had no idea whether such a rule existed. Anyway, he bought the story plus my claim that there were a few more of us kids, each less than 16 years old. So none of us were sent away. I later realized that my chances of survival would have been greater in Siberia than if I were captured by Germany, Russia's great ally at the time.

That alliance lasted less than 2 years. On June 22, 1941, Germany attacked Russia, the day before the anniversary of Napoleon's invasion in 1812. Mirowski tried to enlist in the Russian army but was rejected for being too young, the same reason that the "general" had been led to believe he had no passport. Now he had to flee the advancing German army and continue an odyssey that would cover over 9,000 miles in 4.5 years.

The next stop was Kiev, the great city of the Ukraine on the Dnieper River, where he remembers sleeping in a park. When he and his friends saw officials burning papers, they knew the German army was approaching—the Germans entered Kiev in September 1941—and they continued east. "We tried to take trains. Of course, one never had a ticket and rode both inside and on the roofs of the cars. My daughter once asked me what we ate. I can't really remember. We just ate."

Mirowski settled briefly in Rostov on the Don River just northeast of the Sea of Azov. There he worked on a building crew in the countryside. The next stop was Krasnodar, 150 miles to the south, a quiet town, as he remembers it, with schools for electricians, plumbers, and toolmakers. Krasnodar, under its former name of Ekaterinodar, had been the seat of the White Russian government during the Civil War. The Germans would eventually capture it after much devastation.

Mirowski remembered:

In Krasnodar, I engaged in my first commercial venture, and in communist Russia at that, but this was war time. My friends and I manufactured cigarettes and made some additional money cleaning up at the schools after classes were done. But I heard on the radio that the Germans had taken Rostov and were heading toward Baku. It was time to move east again. One of my friends named Ernst stayed behind with his newly acquired Russian girlfriend who told him they would be safe there. I never saw him again.

East was to Baku—ahead of the Germans—a city important for its oil wells and refineries on the western shore of the Caspian Sea. It was in Baku that Mirowski remembers hearing the Polish national anthem played on the radio in honor of General Sikorski who was raising a Polish army in exile.

Then by ship and train, he traveled through Tashkent to Andijan, an agricultural town in which factories had recently been built presumably beyond the Germans' reach. Mirowski was now over 2,500 miles from Warsaw in a city that lies less than 200 miles from India and Afghanistan to the south and China to the east. In Andijan, he worked up to 11 hours per day in an airplane factory and thereby made, as he put it "my first contribution to beating the Nazis, and I did it with pleasure. Even though I was gainfully employed and somewhat more comfortable physically, each day was a test in survival. A pickpocket once cut my pocket and took my papers, but not my wallet so I still have some pictures. An honest pickpocket!"

Malnutrition was commonplace throughout Russia at this time. Everything was rationed. Mirowski, along with many others, contracted tropical infections for which little treatment was available. Nevertheless, he went to the public library every day to read books and newspapers. By now, Polish nationals were fighting the Germans in Iran, Palestine, and Italy. He read that Stalin had created the first Polish Communist Army and that it was training at a camp near Moscow, "I was freed from the factory and sent to Moscow to join the army. When I got there and was asked for my nationality, I said 'Jewish'—I should have said Polish—and I was sent back to Andijan."

Mirowski then got a different job working for a traveling group of singers, storytellers, and an orchestra. At first, the work was prosaic; he glued up signs and posters. Within 2 weeks, however, he was made an administrator, and life became somewhat more pleasant. He now had time to study and became, in the terms of that time, relatively rich. He could travel and had more coupons for food. One bread coupon was worth 2 weeks of salary.

In 1944, Mirowski volunteered successfully for the army—this time as a Pole—and became a junior officer in the support forces. He had a heart murmur and, therefore, was not assigned to a fighting branch.

Medical School

By the fall of 1945, Mirowski was back in Poland and registered as a medical student at the University of Gdansk. The war was over, but signs of it were everywhere.

He remembered:

> There was no shortage of cadavers—or soap. I saw the camp near Gdansk where the Germans had converted human corpses into soap, and there was a lot of it still available. Warsaw had been completely destroyed, including its ghetto. None of my family was left; I couldn't even find our old home. Two of my friends had survived, hidden by Poles. Their purpose, however, wasn't heroic; they were handsomely paid for it. Their motivation was pure greed.
>
> I stayed in medical school there for a year but gradually came to believe I had to leave Poland. Many Poles still felt that Hitler hadn't finished the job. I had been a local fighter; now I became a Zionist. After all that had happened and that I had seen, the Jews had to have a country of their own to survive. As far as Poland was concerned, it had become a cemetery for me. I told myself that I would never return.

With a friend who now lives in Paris, Mirowski set off again, this time for Palestine. It was illegal then to emigrate there, but he said somewhat defiantly, "That didn't deter me. For six years I had stretched the law. This was necessary simply to survive the war and seemed justified because so many laws were directed specifically against Jews."

Friends had arranged the transport of Jews through Austria, and Mirowski was preparing to leave for Salzburg when his asthma recurred. This had happened previously, the first time when he left his family in 1939 and fled into Russia, and on two or three other occasions when he was about to cross national borders. He was sufficiently ill to miss the group's departure, but later, acting on his own, he entered Germany on the way to France. In Paris, he lived with a few

surviving former classmates and their relatives. Although it was particularly difficult to travel from France to Palestine, Mirowski managed
to obtain a visa.

He arrived in Tel Aviv in the spring of 1947. His paternal grandfather
had settled there many years previously, and he stayed at the home of his
cousins who found him a job as a shoe salesman. He asserted, "I wanted
to continue my education. I was committed to becoming a doctor, if for
no other reason than to honor my father's last words to me, 'Be a physician, be a Jew.'"

Since there were no medical schools operating in Israel in the early
postwar years, Mirowski decided to return to France and seek admission
there. "Even on the boat going back to France, I didn't know where I
would study. It couldn't be Paris; my friends were there. They weren't
studying, and I needed to be where I would not be distracted." On the
ship, Mirowski met a couple from Lyon. He liked what he heard about
the city, traveled there and entered the medical school in the fall of 1947.
His French was poor, and his English almost nonexistent. He listened to
the lectures and demonstrations in French and studied medical texts in
English as he taught himself both languages.

The French medical schools were greatly overcrowded. Five hundred
students started in his class. There were not enough seats in the
amphitheater. No one knew the professors, and the faculty knew none
of the students. Medical school in France took 7 years and included
some subjects that are taught in the premedical courses at American col-
leges. Contact with patients was limited, and most students graduated
without the clinical clerkships and subinternships, which are typical in
the United States and Great Britain. Most graduates then proceeded to
their permanent jobs. Only the best 10% were appointed to the equiva-
lent of house staff positions to prepare themselves for academic or specialty careers. Mirowski remembered,

> As a student, I had the unusual opportunity of getting to know one of
> the members of the faculty, not well of course. He was Professor Roger
> Froment, a leading cardiologist. In the French system you could start
> specializing even as a student. Of course, this might get you nowhere,
> and you'd wind up a general practitioner in the provinces. Anyway, I
> became a cardiologist, before I became an internist.

Froment's field greatly appealed to Mirowski. He was enchanted by cardiology, and it seemed suitable to his way of thinking. The specialty had become extraordinarily exciting. Cardiac catheterization was being applied to the study of congenital and valvular heart disease. Every case seemed to reveal some new knowledge. Surgery of the heart was now possible. Repair of a few congenital defects had been performed just before the war. At the Johns Hopkins Hospital, pediatrician Helen Taussig and surgeon Alfred Blalock had developed an operation for the "blue babies" afflicted with the congenital defect tetralogy of Fallot, and in 1947, successful operative relief of one of the lesions caused by rheumatic fever was announced. The heart–lung machine would be applied for the first time to the repair of another congenital defect in 1953, the year Mirowski graduated. He also found cardiology, at least in France, satisfying for very practical reasons. "I could learn cardiology independently. In surgery, for example, you had to be part of the system, or you could never operate. All my life I have never been part of the system."

Every medical student was required to write a thesis, which could range from very simple to exceedingly involved. Mirowski reviewed a series of patients from Froment's clinic who had undergone cardiac surgery. Eventually, the paper reached 157 pages.

On graduating, Mirowski had to decide where to take further training and to practice. "I knew I wouldn't be staying in France. I would always be a second-class citizen there. Only in Israel or the United States could someone like me be a first-class citizen."

Postgraduate Training

In January 1954, Mirowski returned to Israel, to a country overpopulated with physicians, many of whom were refugees who had been professors and well-known consultants in Europe before the Nazis. Nevertheless, he found a job in the heart station at Tel Hashomer Hospital. He became first assistant to Dr. Harry Heller, the chief of medicine, whom Mirowski saw as

> very firm, a typical German professor, but every day that we made rounds together was a holiday for me. Heller was smart but very Niet-

zschean and not personally helpful. I think he didn't care much about people. He'd fire someone by putting a letter on his desk. I saw him as a stereotype of the German culture of his time.

Nevertheless, Mirowski described Heller as,

the best internist I ever met.

We used English titles left over from the British occupation—I was known as a registrar [resident in the United States]. Although our books were in English, everyday conversation was usually in Hebrew. Actually one could find a person who spoke almost every European language. Yiddish, of course, competed with Hebrew especially among the patients. Hebrew and service in the army unified the country. Israel was more of a melting pot in the 50's than America had ever been.

In 1958, a physician from the Cardiological Institute in Mexico City visited Mirowski's hospital. As soon as he heard him lecture, Mirowski knew he had to go there. Travel was more complex now since Mirowski had a family. In 1950, as a medical student, he had married the sister of the woman from Lyon whom he had met on the boat from Israel to France 3 years earlier. Their first daughter was born in 1959.

About his Mexican experience, Mirowski said,

The person I really wanted to work with was Enrique Cabrera, the only genius I've ever known. He played the piano like a virtuoso and knew archeology better than many professionals. Cabrera, whose father had been Foreign Minister of Mexico, was already a communist. I heard some of his lectures on Marxism-Leninism and had wild debates with him about the 1956 Sinai war. In 1962, Cabrera went to Cuba; I think he may have lost his job. Soon afterwards he developed a brain tumor, went to Russia for an operation and died. He was still quite young.

Even though Mirowski had not learned Spanish previously, he picked up enough to write his first paper two months after arriving in Mexico City.[6] The time he spent there was exceedingly satisfying, but by 1.5 years, he sought different experiences.

I wanted to know how leading people did their work. To my surprise, I was offered a fellowship with Dr. Helen Taussig at Hopkins, and so we came to Baltimore for the first time. Dr. Taussig gave me 10 days to learn to speak English and then put me to work in her clinic. From 8 to 6 I worked for her; after 6, I did my research. My name was on 14 papers from the 2.5 years with her. I felt then, and have always felt, an internal need to investigate and create. One should enter academics because of the drive to make contributions, not for advancement—although it's nice when it comes.

That period in Baltimore was difficult for the family. They were new to the United States and did not have much money, and Mirowski worked very long schedules. By then, there were three young children. Thus, in 1963, Mirowski returned to Israel. He felt a duty to live there, that leaving Israel would constitute a desertion. At the time, he did not even consider remaining in the United States.

Cardiologist in Israel

For the next 5 years, Mirowski was the sole and, therefore, the chief cardiologist at Asaf Harofeh Hospital, 15 miles from Tel Aviv. Asaf Harofeh is a community hospital and provided him with his own carpeted, air-conditioned office, considerably more generous accommodations than his academic colleagues enjoyed at Israeli teaching hospitals. He did not have a secretary or a typewriter, however, and was not the hospital director's most popular doctor.

I was always asking him for things. He said that if they gave me a typewriter, every other chief would want one—a perfect bureaucratic response. Well if you can't get into the room through the door, you get in through the window. I convinced the librarian to lend me his typewriter and with two of my fingers turned out 18 papers. Once I asked for a leave to finish some research and was told to use vacation time. I am afraid my colleagues didn't have much use for me either, but that didn't matter. One can produce and create anywhere even in the intellectual desert to which I had returned.

In 1966, my old boss, Professor Harry Heller, started having bouts of ventricular tachycardia. He was repeatedly hospitalized and treated with quinidine and procainamide [the leading antiarrhythmic drugs of the time]. My wife asked me why I was so concerned. "Because he will die from it," I told her. And he did, two weeks later while at dinner with his family.

From Heller, Mirowski had learned the virtues of logical thinking, and the first step was to read what was known about sudden death. He

was unaware then of the magnitude of the problem and the ineffective-
ness of contemporary therapy. Coronary care units were then being built
in many hospitals. Conversion of ventricular tachycardia and ventricular fibrillation by countershock and prevention of cardiac arrest by suppression of premature beats were generally accepted forms of therapy.
Preventing sudden death after the patients left the hospital seemed
hopeless, however. The antiarrhythmic drugs then available were relatively ineffective, and no medical, surgical, or electrical method of treatment had been shown to prevent cardiac arrest outside of the hospital.
A few patients could be saved by doctors and nurses in mobile coronary
care units, which operated in a few cities, but unless they reached the
patient soon, treatment failed. Mirowski wondered: how could we have
prevented Heller's death at that time: keep him forever in the CCU, or
follow him around with a defibrillator? Both solutions were obviously
impossible. Implantable pacemakers were then becoming available. So, I
reasoned, let's create a similar kind of implantable device to monitor for
ventricular fibrillation and automatically shock the patient back to
sinus rhythm. Should be simple enough.

> I talked to some cardiologists who knew more about such devices. They
> all told me that debrillators couldn't be miniaturized. In those days, a
> defibrillator weighed 30 to 40 pounds; it was preposterous to reduce it to
> the size of a cigarette box. But I had been challenged by the problem, ini-
> tially because of the death of a man I admired very much, but also because
> people told me it couldn't be done. Thank goodness I wasn't an engineer
> because then I would certainly have realized that the idea was crazy.

Mirowski found himself in an unlikely place to accomplish the
impossible. Israeli medicine was run by the government and the trade
union Histradut, the two organizations that owned the hospitals and
employed the doctors. Asaf Harafeh was a government-run community
hospital. Research was conducted in the university teaching hospitals
and seldom in community hospitals.

> As I saw it, there were three prerequisites to developing the device: the
> concept, technology and funding. I had the concept—strenuously ques-
> tioned by leading cardiologists and engineers—but neither of the other
> two. I was outside the university system and had no access to engineer-
> ing or financial support.

Mirowski concluded that only in the United States could he assemble what was needed to make the defibrillator, the building of which had clearly become an obsession and was to remain the principal goal for the rest of his professional life. He recalls,

> In retrospect, moving back to America was one of the most reckless acts of my life. My compulsion now involved my family which had lived in Israel for the last five years, and we had become quite comfortable. I had job tenure, my own office and, what is available to relatively few Israeli doctors, a flourishing private practice. It isn't easy for physicians to do well financially in Israel, but we were OK. We had a house in Savyon, the Beverly Hills of Israel, two cars and a full-time maid.

Mirowski was better known in the United States than where he lived. He usually published in American medical journals and presented papers at American cardiology meetings. He wrote to some friends in the United States and received several inquiries about staff positions. In the spring of 1968, he flew to San Francisco to attend the annual meeting of the American College of Cardiology and to participate by invitation in a seminar on arrhythmias about which he had written several articles.

There he spoke with the chief of cardiology at Sinai Hospital of Baltimore. Mirowski knew about Sinai. Two of his children had been born there when he was working at Hopkins. Sinai was a successful community hospital, actively supported by the philanthropic Jewish community of Baltimore. It had a close academic affiliation with the Johns Hopkins medical school and had been located across the street from the Johns Hopkins Hospital for many years. Recently, Sinai had moved into new buildings, close to the suburban residential areas where most Baltimore Jews then lived.

The offer letter from Sinai, which traveled slowly by surface mail, arrived in Israel after the Mirowskis had reached Baltimore. He would become director of the coronary care unit (Figure 17-2), and most significantly for him, half of his time would be dedicated to research. Sinai had a dog laboratory and a clinical engineering department plus a sympathetic director of medicine in Dr. Albert Mendeloff, who assured Mirowski of the time and support needed for his work. Mirowski, who greatly admired Mendeloff, said, "Al and I never had a contract. I still don't have one with the hospital. Our deal was simple; if things didn't work out, I'd leave."

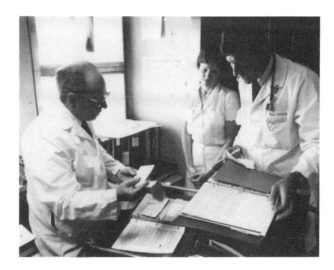

FIGURE 17-2   Michel Mirowski in the Coronary Care Unit at Sinai Hospital of Baltimore

We sold what we owned and after the taxes cleared $6,000 to start our new life. Don't let me overdramatize the move. My wife and eldest daughter had fond memories of the United States and were not unhappy to return. Of course in my unreasonably optimistic way, I knew that this was the right move. America was the only place to do what I wanted to do. Although I might meet hostility there also, and some people were bound to say that my idea was nonsense, you still had a chance to succeed. I couldn't have done it in Israel, France, Britain or Russia.

Back in Baltimore

On September 3, 1968, Michel Mirowski, his wife Anna, and their three children, Ginat (9), Ariella (7), and Doris (6), returned to Baltimore. They rented a house in a northwest suburb of the city, and the children entered the local schools. Mirowski was 44 years old as he and his family began their second life in America. At last, he had found security and professional opportunity after years of flight and turmoil.

By the time he moved to Baltimore, Mirowski had written or was the co-author of 29 articles published in leading American, European,

Israeli, and Mexican medical journals. Most of those on which he was the principal investigator reported clinical studies on electrocardiography and cardiac arrhythmias. Research was really what Mirowski admired. "The creators, of whatever stripe, are my heroes. Recognition by peers, compensation, praise are secondary."

From his earliest days, Mirowski wanted to be a scientist, not the practitioner his father had in mind for him. "There is nothing wrong with practice, or for that matter with being a musician or whatever, but they're not for me." In research, one has no guarantee that the project will succeed, so the investigator must keep his spirits up. Mirowski strongly believed this and recalled a favorite barnyard fable on this point he enjoyed telling his daughters. Two children are together in a room. One is an optimist, the other a pessimist. One of them sniffs the air and says, "I smell horse manure." The optimistic child says, "I think there's a horse outside." Mirowski concluded, "I would always dream about the horse rather than smell the manure."

On first appearance, Sinai Hospital of Baltimore would not seem to be the ideal place for Mirowski to accomplish the impossible. It was, and remains today, a community hospital, not a primary teaching hospital. "I was always slightly outside the mainstream of academic medicine," Mirowski recognizes. "There are those who are accepted, whose futures are planned, whose promise is appreciated. But that's not me. Nobody nursed me along."

He recalled Dr. Harry Heller, his favorite professor in Israel. It was Heller who, unknowingly, inspired Mirowski to his life's work. Heller had developed ventricular tachycardia and, as Mirowski predicted, died suddenly soon afterward. It was 2 years since Heller's death, and the automatic implantable defibrillator seemed as far from reality in 1968 as when Mirowski swore he would develop a device that could treat the arrhythmia that killed his former chief.

Although comfortably established at a fine hospital and enjoying the strong support of his chief, one vital part of his dream was still missing. For all of Michel Mirowski's creativity and persistence, he is not a particularly avid experimenter. At this point, Mirowski spoke with Dr. Morton M. Mower whom Mirowski had met before arriving at Sinai. Mower, a junior member of the hospital staff, ran the hospital's heart station and was starting a private cardiology practice. Morty Mower, a self-described tinkerer, had led a very different life from the man who was to become his collaborator. He had traveled outside the United States only once while an army medical officer in Germany and had lived in the vicinity of Baltimore for the rest of his 36 years. He had graduated only 7 years previously from the University of Maryland Medical School and then trained in medicine and cardiology at the University of Maryland and Sinai Hospitals.

"'Could I build an automatic implantable defibrillator?' Michel asked me in July 1969," Mower remembers. "Mirowski wasn't the only one to have suggested such a device. I had actually thought about it myself—the idea had crossed my mind—but I had considered the whole thing impractical. Now here it was thrown back at me. I'd better not reject it out-of-hand twice." Mower asked for a day or two to think about the project. He had already decided to work with Mirowski, however, and was elated by the extraordinary coincidence that two people with an identical enthusiasm should find themselves in the same institution.

Designing the Defibrillator

It was almost a year after Mirowski moved to the United States before he discussed his concept of the automatic implantable defibrillator with Mower. During this time, Mirowski recalled,

> I had concluded that one could not miniaturize the conventional bulky defibrillator because of constraints in capacitor technology and the need to deliver enough energy—at least 400 joules—to terminate ventricular fibrillation. Therefore, I formulated a working hypothesis that most of the energy used for external defibrillation is wastefully dissipated in the tissues surrounding the heart. One should be able to significantly reduce the energy needed for defibrillation by delivering the shock from within or close to the heart and, consequently, reduce the size of the capacitor sufficiently to build a device suitable for implantation in man. I believe that this initially purely theoretical concept of internal defibrillation in closed chest subjects was the crucial breakthrough which allowed the development of the implantable defibrillator.

For their first experiment, Mower inserted a plate from a broken defibrillator paddle subcutaneously into the chest wall of a dog. A catheter, threaded into the dog's superior vena cava, the great vein that drains the blood from the head and the arms, was used for the other electrode. They then fibrillated the dog's heart with an electric current and successfully converted it with the first shock of 20 joules. This was early in August 1969 and less than 1 month since Mirowski and Mower had begun work-ing together. An auspicious beginning, but their first patient would not be treated for 11 years (Figure 17-3).

Mirowski and Mower decided that they had something specific to report, and they published their first experiences in a general medical journal in 1970.[7] They were not, however, entirely prepared for the diffi-culty that they then encountered securing acceptance for their early work in the cardiology literature. The reviewers were very critical of their manuscripts. "I had always looked on reviewers as helpful by giving instructive criticism to improve the manuscript," Mower says, but in the early 1970s, that is not how they appeared to Mirowski and Mower.

Mirowski said,

> Everybody thought it unfeasible. Someone actually called it a "bomb inside the body." I remember a successful inventor in the pacemaker field who asked me, "Do you know why a defibrillator is so large? It's because you must store energy in capacitors, and to store 400 joules, you'll need capacitors at least 4 inches in each dimension."

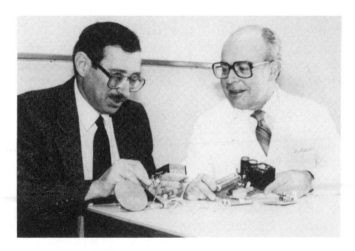

FIGURE 17-3   Drs. Michel Mirowski (right) and Morton Mower reminisce about the events of 1969 with the first working breadboard model of an auto-matic implantable cardioverter defibrillator developed for use in dogs. This photograph was taken in 1985.

Mirowski and Mower never resolved their colleague's objections. Because their device defibrillated inside the chest rather than externally through the chest wall, much less power was needed, and smaller capacitors could be used.

In retrospect, Mirowski and Mower see the rejection of their work during the early 1970s as useful. Many of the objections were helpful and drove the investigators to find solutions that they might not otherwise have emphasized, and the general skepticism kept others out of the field. "There was virtually no competition," Mirowski recalled, but consequently, there were no others working in the area with whom Mirowski and Mower could discuss their problems.

Financing the Work

Furthermore, the unconventional nature of the device and the reservations of consultants precluded Mirowski and Mower's obtaining money from the usual federal and foundation sources. Because funding was unavailable, Mirowski and Mower had to support their work from their own limited resources. Frequently, unconventional solutions were needed, such as obtaining experimental animals directly from the pound at $1.00 per dog. Mower observes that, as could be anticipated by those who know Mirowski,

> Michel shows his badge of "No Grants Asked for or Received" with some pride. At times of adversity, Michel's logical mind gives way. Many of his vital decisions have been illogical, even reckless. The word "No" is not in his vocabulary.

Mower remembers Mirowski frequently saying, "It's not that it can't be done; you haven't found a way to do it. It's a question of mind, not facts."

Constructing further models of their defibrillator required Mirowski and Mower to seek additional collaboration. In the spring of 1970, about 1.5 years after Mirowski had moved back to the United States, a senior officer from a leading pacemaker firm visited the laboratory for a demonstration. After a dog with an early model of the defibrillator had been resuscitated, he asked what would happen if the device had not worked. "So we disconnected the defibrillator and refibrillated the animal," Mower recalls. "The dog died, of course. The executive was impressed."

As the pacemaker company continued with its experiments, Mirowski and Mower came to feel that, as Mower puts it, "They weren't moving fast enough." The company had conducted a marketing survey that convinced them that "few doctors had an interest in an implanted defibrillator or even in sudden death. Michel and I felt that a realization of the need by M.D.s had to be created. The company decided we weren't worth the effort, and we parted. Michel got his patent rights back."

The pair considered forming their own company, but in the meantime, a mutual friend introduced Mirowski to Dr. Stephen Heilman at a conference in Singapore in 1972. Heilman, a physician turned engineer, had formed a small company called Medrad in Pittsburgh. Mower describes it as "a garage-type enterprise, but even then the world's largest supplier of angiographic injectors." The firm had several innovative engineers who could help solve the technical problems that plagued the project at this time.

Animal Studies, the Film

By 1975, the team had built a model that was small enough to be completely implanted in dogs. They had also by now been able to publish a few descriptions of their work as investigators and clinicians became more aware of the importance of sudden cardiac death. Mirowski and Mower remembered how the demonstration of an earlier unimplanted unit had impressed the pacemaker company executive. So, they made a movie, a silent movie, that showed a dog equipped with both the defibrillator and a coil attached to the heart through which a fibrillating current could be transmitted from the surface of the skin. The humans seen in this production are Mower, hobbling across the screen with a cane because of knee injuries from skiing, and Mirowski.

The dog, a healthy appearing mongrel, stood still as the inducer was placed on the coil. The animal's heart fibrillated; cardiac output disappeared, and in a few seconds, the dog lost consciousness. The defibrillator sensed the loss of normal cardiac electrical activity and charged the capacitors. The dog was next seen to shudder slightly as the device discharged and in a few more seconds was standing again.

When they first showed the film, "A wag in one of our audiences asked if the dog had been trained to do what we filmed—in some Pavlovian way," Mower recalls. So they added the dog's electrocardiogram along the bottom of the film synchronized to the action. The arrhythmia and the conversion could be clearly correlated with the dog's collapse and recovery. This touch of Hollywood proved to be extraordinarily persuasive. Mirowski and Mower showed it on the increasing number of occasions when they were invited to speak about their work.

Ready for Humans

Soon thereafter, the group converted the canine unit into a device suitable for human implantation. Its hermetic seal was improved, and toxicity tests were conducted. Defibrillators were installed chronically in 25 dogs that survived an average of 3 years.[12] About every 3 months, the dogs were fibrillated, and the device was discharged.

Mirowski and Mower were then ready to implant their first unit in a patient. For this step, they went to the Johns Hopkins Hospital because Sinai Hospital had no cardiac surgical program. At Hopkins, Dr. Myron Weisfeldt, the chief of cardiology, and Dr. Philip Reed, the clinical electrophysiologist, helped guide the device through the Hopkins institutional review board. After approval was obtained, the first patient was treated successfully in February 1980.[3,13]

During the next 5 years, the automatic implantable defibrillator (AID) was installed in 800 patients in several university hospitals. Mower says,

> For our first 50 patients, the mortality from arrhythmias was less than 10%. It would have been 40% to 50% in the patients we treated if they hadn't received the device. The FDA was very cooperative during the premarket clinical trial. We wanted to be more Catholic than the Pope and would do even more than the FDA wanted.

The FDA encouraged Mirowski and Mower to seek full approval before the developers actually wanted to do so. "We would have preferred more pre-market testing," recalls Mower. They were worried about the clinical results at hospitals where they could no longer exercise close control. "It would be easier to keep track of 2,000 rather than 50,000 devices."

With release of the AID from clinical trials, demand for the units increased rapidly and quickly surpassed the manufacturing capacity of Medrad, the "garage-type enterprise," which had developed and pro-duced the earlier units. In 1985, Medrad assigned all its rights and knowledge about the defibrillator to CPI, an established pacemaker company and a division of Eli Lilly since the 1970s.

With the AID becoming an accepted method of treatment, Mirowski's and Mower's roles changed from developers to refiners. The automatic implantable defibrillator became the automatic implantable cardioverter-defibrillator that could detect ventricular tachycardia as well as ventricular fibrillation and cardiovert as well as defibrillate. The weight of the devices decreased from 225 grams in 1980 to 90 grams in 1998 and the size over the same period from 250 to 48 cubic centime-ters. Models using electrode-catheters rather than myocardial patches and, therefore, implantable like pacemakers with local anesthesia and no thoracotomy were developed and have now become standard. Mirowski has been proved correct here as well. "We're smart people, but we don't pretend to know everything," Mower acknowledges. (One can hear Mirowski making the same statement as well.) "There comes a cer-tain point in time when no one can louse it up. So the 'child' left its par-ents. We knew it was in good hands, and we'd continue to have a role as consultants."

Mirowski's and Mower's prediction that their "child" would shrink further as even smaller batteries, capacitors, and inductors were devel-oped came to pass. Software replaced hardware so that current devices perform more specialized functions such as detecting a wider range of arrhythmias and converting by pacing as well as by shock. Physicians can now program transcutaneously many features of the device's sens-ing and discharging functions.

By the end of 2005, more than a million units, it is estimated, had been implanted worldwide. As Mirowski and Mower predicted,[14] physi-cians now implant cardioverter-defibrillators prophylactically in patients who have not as yet suffered from ventricular tachycardia and fibrillation but are at high risk of developing these arrhythmias.

Illness

In the mid 1980s, Mirowski became ill. In retrospect, his family believes that the first symptoms appeared while the family was vacationing at a beach. Using her father as the subject, Ariella was demonstrating the chest examination to Doris. She touched him in the ribs, a tap that should not have hurt as much as it did. In typical fashion, he medicated himself for the pain, which gradually became severe. Finally, he agreed to be admitted to Johns Hopkins Hospital, and multiple myeloma, a cancer of one of the elements of the blood, was diagnosed. Treatment relieved his symptoms for several years. However, in 1989, a more virulent leukemia developed. He insisted on receiving the most intensive chemotherapy, fighting against the odds as usual. When the disease stopped responding, his oncologist raised the possibility of a bone-marrow transplant, then in experimental development for the treatment of myeloma. A near relative as donor would be needed. Did he have a brother? This would have been Abraham, lost in the Holocaust. When Mirowski died on March 26, 1990, at the age of 65 years, he had more than 20 pathological fractures.

For years, but particularly during his final illness, Mirowski was tortured by regret that he had not adequately honored the name of his parents. (On becoming an American citizen, he had officially adopted the name, Michel Mirowski.) He ordered that his gravestone read as follows: "Michel Mirowski son of Israel Lieb Friedman and Genia Handelsman."

Family and Reputation

In his 60s, by then a leading figure in international cardiology, Mirowski appeared as a man of his years, of medium height, slightly overweight with thinning gray hair, and the demeanor of a scholar. His speech was highly articulate, laced with classical and literary references. A listener was always surprised when Mirowski could not find the precisely correct English word to express what he wished to say. He would then recall the *mot juste* in some other language. Mirowski's English had a slight accent, clearly European but difficult for the American ear to localize further. Always wanting to know what was happening everywhere, he compulsively read *The New York Times* every day and was clearly uneasy until his copy arrived.

Anna, his wife for 40 years, continued to maintain a European ambiance in their Baltimore home. She projected warmth and sensitivity with an elegance and formality of speech and manner from her European background. Food always mattered to Anna and Michel Mirowski, but probably for different reasons. Michel observed from less happy times that fat people survive. So one should eat a lot, and Mirowski, more than his wife, was likely to offer the second helping. Of the two, however, Anna Mirowski is the more practical and the more sentimental. When she talked about him, Mirowski was always "my Michel" or "my dear Michel." She claimed that she started using this title to distinguish her Michel from another Michel, also a refugee in Lyons. Anna Mirowski died in 2001.

Each of Anna and Michel's daughters are now physicians. Mirowski insisted that he "bent over backward" not to push his children into medical careers. "I tried to be supportive but neutral. The worst way to get them to do something is to tell them to do it." When his children complained about their work, Mirowski liked to respond, "The bumps in the road are not bumps, they are the road. You're not being punished; you do it because you want to." Anna, however, encouraged the children to be doctors almost from infancy. She wanted them to have professions, "not be just a housewife like me," and she had observed that doctors usually prospered even in difficult times because of the value of their work. The names of their children honor Michel and other members of the Mirowski and their husbands' families.

The last 5 years of his life brought Mirowski the recognition that was not his in earlier times. Professional societies and leaders of academic medical institutions honored him. He received invitations to write more articles and give more lectures than he could accept. Thus, he picked and chose, accommodating his friends and those who supported him in darker times. Often with his wife or children he traveled where he wished because now he was welcome everywhere.

When he spoke overseas, Mirowski usually lectured in English, but he often discussed his papers during the question-and-answer period in the language of the country that he was visiting. He spoke French, Hebrew, Polish, Russian, Spanish, and Yiddish fluently, but he never learned Italian and would not learn German. Some things cannot be forgotten.

Chapter 18

Wolff, Parkinson, and White

The three names associated with the Wolff-Parkinson-White syndrome were all doctors specializing in cardiology in the early 1930s when the field was young (Figure 18-1). Paul Dudley White, who worked at the Massachusetts General Hospital (MGH) in Boston, had been collecting examples of abnormal electrocardiograms of otherwise healthy young people with tachycardia for several years and had discussed the cases with the English cardiologist John Parkinson. During the year that Louis Wolff was a trainee in White's department, Parkinson and White decided to report the cases and assigned Wolff to write the first draft. Of the 11 cases reported, seven came from London and four from Boston.[12] In August, 1930, the article first describing the syndrome appeared in the *American Heart Journal*, then the principal journal in which American doctors published research in cardiology.[13]

When they reported the cases, the authors knew little about the mechanisms involved. They concluded, mistakenly, that the abnormality of the QRS complex—a slurring at its onset, called a *delta wave*—reflected bundle branch block in which part of the conducting tissue transmitting the signal from atria to ventricles malfunctions. The short P-R interval baffled them. Furthermore, they could not explain how the

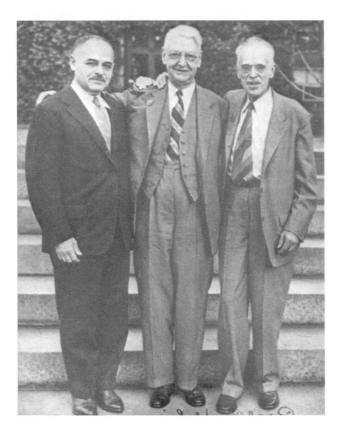

FIGURE 18-1   Dr. Louis Wolff (left), Sir John Parkinson (middle), and Dr. Paul Dudley White (right) during Parkinson's visit to Boston in 1954 when the English cardiologist met his co-author Louis Wolff for the first time. They are standing on the stone steps in front of the Bulfinch Building, the original structure of MGH where White worked throughout his distinguished career. The informality among these famous collaborators is striking—arms on shoulders, Parkinson's vest unbuttoned. The Parkinson-White professional and personal friendship lasted for more than 60 years.

abnormal electrocardiogram accounted for the tachycardia, the principal clinical manifestation of the syndrome.

Two of the three authors were among the founders of the specialty of cardiology, White in the United States and Parkinson in Britain. Paul Dudley White (1886–1973), the son of a family doctor in Roxbury, Massachusetts, graduated from Harvard College and its medical school (MD

1911) and trained in internal medicine at the MGH. Just before the beginning of the First World War, in which he served as a doctor, White spent a year learning the new technique of electrocardiography with Thomas (later Sir Thomas) Lewis at University College Hospital in London. On returning to Boston after the war, White established, in 1919, the cardiac unit at the MGH, one of the first in the country. In 1931, the year after the Wolff-Parkinson-White syndrome was described, he published the first of four editions of his text *Heart Disease*, which quickly became a standard work on the subject.[14]

After relinquishing leadership of the cardiac unit in 1949, the division that he had founded 3 decades earlier, White became increasingly involved in international cardiology, traveling frequently to many countries. The general public first learned of him as a consultant to President Dwight Eisenhower during his myocardial infarction in 1955. Typical of this New England doctor, White's news conferences included much more detail about his patient's medical condition than was then customarily revealed by the doctor of a well-known figure such as the president.[15] The second activity, which brought him renown, was his custom of bicycle riding even in his later years to emphasize the wisdom of keeping fit. The 17-mile Dr. Paul Dudley White Bike Path in the Boston-Brookline area is named for him. White continued seeing patients until felled by a cerebral hemorrhage (stroke), to which he succumbed at the age of 87 years, at the MGH, of course.

Sir John Parkinson (1885–1976, knighted in 1948), "the best known and most influential British cardiologist of the second quarter of the 20th century," according to his biographer,[16] earned his medical degrees from the University of London.[17] He was long associated with the London Hospital, where he directed its cardiac department and with the National Heart Hospital. Parkinson had met White in 1913 when the American was training in London.

After his training with White, Louis Wolff (1898–1972), who like White, was a graduate of the Harvard Medical School, joined the staff of the Beth Israel Hospital, one of the Harvard teaching hospitals in Boston, where he practiced cardiology and directed the electrocardiography laboratory.

During the 1930s, several investigators tried to explain the origin of the electrocardiographic abnormalities in the Wolff-Parkinson-White syndrome and why these patients have tachycardias. The most convincing hypothesis proposed that an *accessory pathway* could account for the short P-R interval, the delta waves, and the tendency for patients with the Wolff-Parkinson-White syndrome to develop tachycardia.

Then, in 1943, Francis Wood, working in the cardiology unit led by Charles Wolferth at the University of Pennsylvania, reported finding an abnormal "muscular connection" between the atria and ventricles during an autopsy on the heart of a patient who had had the Wolff-Parkinson-White syndrome in life.* Wood and Wolferth, as well as other investigators before them, had postulated that the P-R interval should be shorter than normal if the accessory pathway could conduct intracardiac signals from atria to ventricles faster than could the normal pathway within the atioventricular node and bundle of His.

The insertion of the accessory pathway into the ventricles at a location distant from the insertion of the normal conduction tissues could explain the delta wave as a reflection of early abnormal activation of the ventricles from the eccentric termination of the accessory pathway. Wood and Wolferth also suggested that the tachycardias might be "initiated by retrograde [ventricles to atria] conduction, through the accessory tract, of an excitatory process which had previously been transmitted to the ventricles via the normal channels."[18] Each of the hypotheses put forward by Wood and Wolferth would later be proven correct.

Charles Wolferth, a clinical investigator with strong opinions, eschewed using the eponym Wolff-Parkinson-White syndrome, which appeared nowhere in the text of the 1943 article even though, by then, the phrase had entered the medical lexicon of many cardiologists.[18] Wolferth preferred to call the condition "short P-R interval and prolonged QRS complex."[18] He also employed the word "preexcitation," which emphasized premature activation of the ventricles as the primary abnormality. Regardless of the nomenclature used, Wood and Wolferth's discovery provided attractive explanations for the abnormal electrocardiograms and tachycardias in these patients. Later studies would explain more fully how the accessory pathway participates in and sustains the arrhythmias characteristic of the syndrome.

---

* These accessory pathways are sometimes called *Kent bundles* in honor of Stanley Kent who first demonstrated them in humans and animals.

References

1. White PD. *Heart Disease*. 4th ed. New York: Macmillan Company; 1951:900.
2. Gould WL. Auricular fibrillation. *Archives of Internal Medicine* 1957;100:916–926.
3. Koskinen P, Kupari M, Leinonen H. Role of alcohol in recurrences of atrial fibrillation in persons less than 65 years of age. *American Journal of Cardiology* 1990;66:954–958.
4. Andrew Rosenthal. Bush's physicians say thyroid gland disrupted heart. *New York Times*. May 8, 1991:A1.
5. Luria MH. Selected clinical features of paroxysmal tachycardia: a prospective study of 20 patients. *British Heart Journal* 1971;33:351–357.
6. Parkinson J, Bedford D. The course and treatment of auricular flutter. *Quarterly Journal of Medicine* 1927;21:21–50.
7. Waldo AL. Atrial flutter. In: Podrid P, Kowey P, eds. *Cardiac Arrhythmia. Mechanism, diagnosis and management*. Baltimore: Williams & Wilkins; 1995:791.
8. Shine KI, Kastor JA, Yurchak PM. Multifocal atrial tachycardia. Clinical and electrocardiographic features in 32 patients. *New England Journal of Medicine* 1968;279:344–349.

9. Anonymous. *Paul Wood's Diseases of the Heart and Circulation*. 3rd ed. Philadelphia: J.B. Lippincott Company; 1968:245.

10. Hurst JW. Naming of the waves in the ECG, with a brief account of their genesis. *Circulation* 1998;98:1937–1942.

11. Kastor JA. Michel Mirowski and the implantable cardioverter defibrillator. In: *Arrhythmias*. 2nd ed. Philadelphia: W. B. Saunders; 2000:23–34.

12. Wolff L. Wolff-Parkinson-White syndrome: historical and clinical features. *Progress in cardiovascular disease* 1960;2:677–690.

13. Wolff L, Parkinson J, White PD. Bundle-branch block with short P-R interval in healthy young people prone to paroxysmal tachycardia. *American Heart Journal* 1930;5:685–704.

14. White PD. *Heart Disease*. First edition. New York: Macmillan Company, 1931.

15. Lasby CG. *Eisenhower's heart attack. How Ike beat heart disease and held on to the presidency*. Lawrence, Kansas: University Press of Kansas, 1997:86–88.

16. Bauer GE. Sir John Parkinson 1885–1976. In: Silverman ME, Fleming PR, Hollman A, Julian DG, Krikler DM, eds. *British Cardiology in the 20th Century*. London: Springer-Verlag London Limited; 2000:370–373.

17. John Parkinson. *Lancet* 1976;1:1536.

18. Wood FA, Wolferth GC, Geckeler GD. Histological demonstration of accessory muscular connection between auricle and ventricle in a case of short P-R interval and prolonged QRS complex. *American Heart Journal* 1943;25:454–462.

Index